WU100 JUN

D0297506

54008000069557

Emergencies in Dental Practice
Diagnosis and Management

Emergencies in Dental Practice
Diagnosis and Management

RICHARD P. JUNIPER
BRIAN J. PARKINS

and contribution from

A. J. RODESANO
Consultant Orthodontist, John Radcliffe Hospital

HEINEMANN MEDICAL BOOKS

Heinemann Medical Books
An imprint of Heinemann Professional Publishing Ltd
Halley Court, Jordan Hill, Oxford OX2 8EJ

OXFORD LONDON SINGAPORE NAIROBI IBADAN KINGSTON

First published 1990

© R. P. Juniper and B. J. Parkins 1990

ISBN 433–02266–3

British Library Cataloguing in Publication Data
Juniper, Richard
  Emergencies in dental practice.
  1. Dentistry. Emergency treatment
  I. Title   II. Parkins, B. J.
  617.6026

Typeset by Lasertext, Stretford, Manchester
and printed in Great Britain by
Redwood Press Ltd
Melksham, Wilts

Contents

	Preface	vii
1.	Facial Pain	1
2.	Acute Swellings Related to Dental Tissues	15
3.	Trauma	26
4.	Haemorrhage from the Mouth	35
5.	Emergencies Involving the Oral Mucous Membrane	40
6.	Medical Emergencies	55
7.	Management of HIV and Hepatitis B (HBV) Patients	70
8.	The Dentist's Responsibility in Cases of Suspected Child Abuse	72
9.	Restorative Emergencies	76
10.	Endodontic Emergencies	87
11.	Periodontal Emergencies	94
12.	Prosthodontic Emergencies	99
13.	Orthodontic Emergencies	106
14.	Misadventures in the Surgery	109
15.	Emergency Hospital Management of Facial Pain	119
16.	Emergency Hospital Management of Acute Swellings	128
17.	Emergency Hospital Management of Trauma	133
18.	Emergency Hospital Management of Haemorrhage	150
19.	Emergency Hospital Management of Acute Conditions of the Oral Mucous Membranes	154
20.	Sedation Emergencies in Practice and Hospital	158
	Appendix	164
	Index	166

Preface

It is anticipated that this little book will find a place in every dental surgery, and in the pocket of every dental house officer. Emergencies happen infrequently and most dental practitioners will hope that there will be none in his/her practising lifetime. However, no matter how careful, how conscientious and how efficient a practitioner is, emergencies and accidents do happen. The sudden and unexpected event leaves most people wondering what they should do, and an inertia bordering on panic may set in. Probably it is the most scrupulous practitioner who is most deeply affected, for he has not been faced with the serious and unexpected before. During emergencies however, there is little time to think and, with turmoil all around, the brain ceases to function efficiently – or at all. It is in these moments that we hope that this publication will be invaluable.

The book is in two sections. The first and major one is directed towards general dental practice, and deals with emergencies which may occur there. The emergencies are tabulated as chapters and will be found most easily in the front of the book although an index is available at the back where more detail will be found. The text is prepared in an easily-read form so that the information may be assimilated in the shortest possible time. Subjects range from the fractured dental restoration and uncontrolled haemorrhage, through to medical emergencies such as diabetic coma and cardiac arrest.

The second section has been prepared for the newly-qualified practitioner who has been appointed dental house officer at a busy accident centre. It is expected that this book will be particularly helpful to such a person who, though inexperienced, will be faced with emergency referrals from more experienced colleagues, who may telephone initially for advice and then ask that the houseman take over management of the case. The first section of the book could prove invaluable during that telephone conversation and early treatment of the case, while the second should prove helpful when the patient has arrived at hospital and further management is required. Definitive treatment of the serious case is not considered as it is expected that more senior staff will be available to take over the management.

1: Facial Pain

To treat facial pain effectively it is first essential to make a correct diagnosis. Approximately 50% of facial pains are straightforward to diagnose, a further 30% are less easy, while 20% require a detailed and systematic approach to reach a correct conclusion. By taking a careful history (*see* Table 1.1), and spending two or three minutes discussing the pain with the patient, most facial pains can be diagnosed with confidence and accuracy.

METHODS OF INVESTIGATION

1. History

Character of the pain: sharp or dull. There are predominantly two main pains, a sharp pain as if a needle is being plunged into the skin or a dull pain like toothache which is continuous. Sharp pains last a maximum of five seconds, but are usually of even shorter duration, while dull pains last hours or days and may throb. For instance a throbbing pain of a severe nature is indicative of pulpal necrosis. This pain increases to a climax and may abate with the appearance of a swelling.

Patients may wish to describe other pains, but generally can be guided towards one of these two. A burning pain for instance, described for glossodynia, can be looked upon as a continuous pain, while a burning pain experienced with trigeminal neuralgia usually has a character of 'pins and needles', a repetitive sharp pain. Close questioning of the patient will differentiate the two. This separation of pain into two groups is a vital start to the history.

Table 1.1 Facial pain — essential points in a history

Character of the pain – sharp or dull
Site (unilateral, bilateral or crossing the midline)
Duration
Timing
Exacerbating factors
Relieving factors: response to analgesics
Effects on sleep

Site: unilateral, bilateral or crossing the midline. Where possible persuade the patient to point with one finger to the site of the pain, tracing it over the area if it covers more than the size of the finger tip. If it is a dull pain, try to get the patient to identify the prime site and source. Pains arising from pathology are exclusively unilateral with the exception of sinusitis, while those which migrate from one side of the face to the other and can be traced across the anterior midline are generally suggestive of a psychological overlay.

If the character and site of the pain are clarified at the outset, as can be seen from Table 1.2, the possible diagnoses are already being grouped. There are only three causes of sharp pain and they are all unilateral. There are only three dull pains which are bilateral.

Duration. The duration of sharp pain is never more than a few seconds. If a patient insists that their sharp pain lasts longer, it may mean that it represents repetitive sharp pain with transitory painless intervals, or is in reality a dull pain but felt severely. Dull pain may last from minutes to weeks.

It is important to determine the duration of the pain early in the history. For example, the pain of periodic migranous neuralgia seldom lasts more than two hours, while that of atypical facial pain may last weeks, yet both may be felt in the same area.

Timing. Defining the time when the pain begins or is at its worst, again is important. A dull pain over the ramus of the mandible after chewing or talking, suggests TM joint dysfunction, while that after an argument at work may suggest atypical facial pain.

Table 1.2   Facial pain — a scheme for diagnosis

	Unilateral	Bilateral
Exposed dentine, early pulpitis	Sharp	○
Paroxysmal trigeminal neuralgia	Sharp	○
Glossopharyngeal neuralgia	Sharp	○
Toothache – pulpitis or periodontitis	Dull	○
TM Joint dysfunction	Dull	○
Periodic migranous neuralgia	Dull	○
Herpes zoster	Dull	○
Cranial arteritis	Dull	○
Tumours	Dull	○
Sinusitis	○	Dull
Atypical facial pain	○	Dull
Atypical odontalgia	○	Dull

Exacerbating factors. Reaction to heat and sweetness, suggests pulpal involvement while pain in the midface on bending and jarring suggests sinusitis. Throbbing pain which is exacerbated when lying down or walking suggests acute inflammation. Pain on biting suggests a cracked tooth or one which is periodontally involved. This may be evident especially in teeth which have been heavily restored. A similar complaint may be present if a crown or part of a fixed bridge has become uncemented. Pain which is experienced on touching the face lightly suggests trigeminal neuralgia.

Relieving factors: response to analgesics. Sharp pains do not respond to analgesics but generally dull pains do. A dull pain which is not affected by analgesics suggest atypical facial pain or atypical odontalgia. Pain relieved by biting suggests a periodontal origin or early pulpitis.

Effects on sleep. Sharp pain, except that caused by pulpitis, almost never affects sleep although a patient may wake from other causes and then feel the sharp pain. Organic dull pain almost always affects sleep but mercifully is reduced by analgesics. Atypical facial pain although severe in the daytime, never affects sleep.

2. Clinical examination

The clinical examination must be closely related to the findings made from the patient's history. Ideally it confirms the preconceived suspicions of the diagnostician.

3. Special tests

The special tests, for example radiographs, electric pulp testing, and transillumination have to be relevant to the condition being considered to confirm the preliminary diagnosis already made from the history and clinical examination. Special tests are mentioned in the relevant sections relating to specific problems.

FACIAL PAINS AND THEIR MANAGEMENT

A useful and convenient method of considering facial pains is by classifying them as sharp or dull, unilateral or bilateral (*see* Table 1.2). This classification must only be considered as a guide because some conditions, eg pulpitis, atypical facial pain, atypical odontalgia and sinusitis may not always present or progress along these strict confines.

I UNILATERAL SHARP PAIN

Pain of *dental origin* may arise from the pulp (reversible or irreversible pulpitis), the periodontal supporting tissues or from both. The patient complains of *toothache*. This may start as a sharp pain, which becomes dull and unless it is associated with anterior teeth, does not cross the midline.

Pulpitis may present as *reversible pulpitis* or *irreversible pulpitis*. These terms describe the clinical and histopathological presentation of the condition. A patient who has a pulp which is causing a problem may give a bizarre clinical history which does not appear to fit into either of the categories of pulpal pathology described here.

There is no real line of differentiation to guide the clinician in correctly diagnosing the histological state of the pulp tissue which is causing a problem. The only practical necessity is to decide if the pulpitis is irreversible because once this diagnosis has been made the management is the same. The more common clinical features will be described in the relevant sections of the text.

Reversible pulpitis

This is characterized by a sharp pain of very short duration which does not linger on removal of the stimulus and which is difficult to localize. The tooth is not tender to percussion and gives exaggerated response to vitality tests. Radiographs usually show no apparent change (see also page 6 and 7).

Irreversible pulpitis

The management is described on page 6–9.

Paroxysmal trigeminal neuralgia

This is a sharp pain lasting for seconds only, felt in the face, most commonly in the second and third divisions of the trigeminal nerve. It never crosses the midline and infrequently crosses from one division to another in an individual bout. Identification of the division is important for treatment purposes. The condition generally occurs in the over 50's, but can occur earlier and is slightly more common in females than males. In the severest form it is incapacitating with the patients living in fear of the next paroxysm.

Classically there are trigger points, where touching or brushing a certain part of the face may initiate pain. The pain comes as a series of sharp jabs, each lasting less than one second but may repeat rapidly over minutes. It is noted for its exacerbations and remissions and thus may seem to respond to inappropriate remedies. Occasionally an exacerbation may be precipitated by an inflammatory focus such as a dental abscess or TM joint dysfunction.

Emergency treatment Inject local anaesthetic solution, preferably bupivacaine (Marcain) in the region of the appropriate peripheral nerve. For further treatment see Chapter 15.

Glossopharyngeal neuralgia

This is a very uncommon condition identical with paroxysmal trigeminal neuralgia except for the site. Sharp, shooting pain is felt in the throat and tongue, particularly on swallowing. For further treatment see Chapter 15.

II UNILATERAL DULL PAIN

This is a continuous dull pain which can be likened to toothache. A careful history is essential. With a good history and a competent clinician, examination of the patient is needed only to confirm the diagnosis already made.

Pulpitis

This presents as a dull pain, initially fairly well localized, but as the severity and time of suffering increases, it becomes more diffuse. It lasts but a few minutes precipitated by hot, cold and sweet stimuli and may be preceeded by the sharp pain associated with exposed dentine. At each subsequent stimulation the pain lasts longer and may increase in intensity. As the pulpitis progresses, the dull pain progresses. It may start spontaneously and interfere with sleep. The tooth becomes hypersensitive to stimuli and increasingly tender to percussion. It begins to interfere with normal mastication and, as the inflammation spreads through the tissues, the act of bringing the teeth into occlusion becomes painful.

The most common causes of pulpitis are:

1. Caries
2. A fractured restoration
3. A cracked or fractured tooth
4. Iatrogenic causes   (i)   Thermal
                  (ii)   Chemical
                 (iii)   Occlusal
                 (iv)   Orthodontic
5. Exposure of sensitive dentine as a result of gingival recession or erosion, with or without attrition
6. An uncemented restoration especially a bridge retainer
7. Following pulpotomy and pulp capping procedure
8. Advanced Periodontal disease

Irreversible pulpitis which may follow reversible pulpitis, often leads to a *periapical abscess* months or years later. The notable change is that the pain is continuous and is no longer made worse by hot, cold and sweet stimuli. The offending tooth can be identified and becomes increasingly tender to chewing and tapping; bringing the teeth together in the intercuspal position will be very uncomfortable. The pain interferes with sleep but responds well initially to simple analgesics such as aspirin or paracetamol. As the inflammation increases however, these analgesics become less effective, sleep becomes more difficult and pyrexia may develop.

The patient will be unwell, pale from lack of sleep, sweaty from an increased temperature and toxins from the spreading infection. The tooth in question will be exquisitely tender to percussion, extruded slightly from its socket and its gingivae swollen and hyperaemic. Extra-oral palpation will elicit a site of tenderness and the local lymph nodes may be tender.

A radiograph will reveal a widening of the periodontal membrane space in the later stages.

Caries

Management. Remove all carious dentine. Depending on the degree of destruction and integrity of the pulpal tissues and proceed as follows:-

1. Restore the cavity with a properly lined restoration
2. Insert a zinc oxide-eugenol dressing if the cavity is very deep and if there is no clinical evidence of pulpal exposure. Make sure that the patient realizes that this is a provisional restoration which has to be replaced.
3. Carry out pulp capping or pulpotomy procedure using calcium hydroxide sealed in with glass ionomer cement where there is clinical evidence of a small exposure, especially in the teeth of young persons.
4. Root canal therapy is required if there is clinical evidence of an exposure in an adult tooth. Make sure that the patient understands that further treatment will be required to complete the procedure.
5. Extract the tooth if the amount of tooth tissue remaining is unrestorable after all the caries have been removed.

Fractured restoration

Locate the offending restoration by clinical examination. The restoration may be loose or only fractured with one part of it loose. Pressure on the restoration may elicit discomfort and close examination of the margins may reveal the escape of bubbles of saliva.

Management. Remove the offending restoration and proceed as for the carious tooth described above in section on Caries.

Cracked tooth

The patient compains of discomfort on biting which is relieved by separating the occluding teeth. Other symptoms are pain to hot and cold stimuli which may produce anything from mild to intense discomfort. Periods of remission are common.

Management

1. Look for crazing on the surface of the enamel
2. Transilluminate the tooth with a bright light (a fibre optic light or a visible light curing light).
3. Ask the patient to bite on a carefully positioned hard object such as a wood stick.
4. Radiographs should be taken to rule out the presence of other

possible causes but are of little help in diagnosing this problem.

5. Reassure the patient that in time, a piece of the tooth will eventually drop away. This is preferable to breaking off other cusps in an attempt to find the offending one.

6. Remove that part of the tooth which exhibits frank mobility. Assess the involvement of the pulp at this stage.

7. Dress the exposed dentine with calcium hydroxide covered with glass ionomer cement, if the remainder of the tooth if restorable. Commence root canal therapy if there is pulpal involvement.

8. Extract the remainder of the tooth if it is unrestorable

In the case of multi-rooted teeth, where the line of fracture passes along the floor of the pulp chamber and between the roots, consider removing just one of the remaining roots. (*see* Chapter 2, page 34)

Iatrogenic causes

The following should be prevented by awareness of the problems at the time of treatment, however even with the greatest of care, pulp damage may occur from:

1. *Cavity preparation*
   - by not using light intermittent pressure on the bur
   - inadequate cooling of the bur with water
   - overpreparation
   - dessication of the dentine with an air syringe
2. *Chemical irritation*
   - dessication of the dentine by 'cleaning' the cavity with alcohol
   - inadequate pulp protection and poor choice of lining materials

If there is any pulpal discomfort resulting from recent dental treatment, locate the offending tooth by information from the history, and from clinical examination. This usually reveals a recently placed restoration, the integrity of which may be confirmed on an intra-oral radiograph. The restoration may require removal and the ensuing cavity preparation treated following the procedures outlined above in the section on Pulpitis.

3. *Occlusal*: Ensure restorations are not 'high' in all mandibular excursions.

4. *Orthodontics*: Ensure that the orthodontic forces of the spring or arch wire do not produce severe pain. If this should occur, ease the pressure of the activated part of the appliance. If fixed appliances are *in situ*, remove the arch wire and tell the patient

to see the orthodontist as quickly as possible (*see* Chapter 13).

5. *Exposed dentine*: This is a sharp pain. It lasts for seconds only and is well localized. It is precipitated by hot, cold, sweet and citrous foods. The patient can identify the area. It is treated by applying a fluoride varnish in the short-term, or glass ionomer cement or a dentine bonding agent in the longer-term (see also p. 98).

6. *Uncemented bridge retainer*: This may be revealed by exerting pressure over the abutment tooth and observing bubbles of saliva being expressed from the margins of the restoration.

This problem is often associated with 'pier' abutment teeth (ie the middle one of three abutment teeth each separated from the other by a pontic) (*see* also Chapter 9). If the bridge proves to be uncemented:

    (a) Remove bridge and recement (easier said than done but worth a try), or

    (b) Cut the cemented retainer, remove the bridge and recement the damaged bridge as a provisional, or

    (c) Cut off the bridge. Fabricate and cement a provisional bridge.

7. *Following pulp cap or pulpotomy*: If the discomfort is severe, remove the restoration from the tooth and instigate root canal therapy.

8. *Advanced periodontal disease*: Clean and curette the offending area, irrigate with saline and advise the use of a hot saline mouthwash hourly. Prescribe antibiotics if there is a pyrexia. Treat a localized periodontal abscess by establishing drainage, irrigation, curettage as far as possible and advise the patient to use hourly hot mouth washes. Ensure that the patient is seen on a subsequent appointment for recontouring of the gingival architecture.

TM joint dysfunction

This produces a predominantly unilateral dull pain around the ear and side of the face, frequently confused by the patient as earache. Further questioning may reveal that it is bilateral, with one side much more severe than the other. It occurs at almost any age but is more frequently seen in the 15–25 age group with a second lesser group of 35–50. The male/female ratio ranges between 1:5 and 1:9.

The condition is characterized by pain in and around the ear, restricted opening of the mouth and noise in the joint. Initially the pain may be around the joint itself, predominantly on opening, protrusion and heavy chewing, but in acute and severe forms the pain may be felt over the side of the face, head and occasionally in the neck. A diagnosis is made by finding tenderness over the lateral pole of the condyle and in the masseter muscle, particularly the posterior fibres below the condyle. There may be deviation of the mouth on opening.

Management. In the acute phase aspirin, paracetamol or a non-steroidal anti-inflammatory agent such as ibuprofen (400 mg six hourly) are helpful. Some find relief from an occlusal splint which prevents the teeth from reaching the intercuspal position. Advise the patient to take a soft diet, avoid prostrusive movements of the mandible, particularly that of incising, and opening the mouth widely.

An auriculotemporal block using lignocaine or bupivacaine will relieve the pain but runs the risk of temporary facial paralysis necessitating an eye patch. Corticosteroids injected into the joint itself should *never* be used because they may permanently damage the joint. Subsequent treatment is directed to the cause. For further treatment *see* Chapter 15.

Periodic migranous neuralgia (cluster headache)

This condition affects any age group and both sexes but is predominant in the 20–50 age group. It does occur in the elderly. It is characterized by a dull, severe, unilateral pain usually felt in the midface spreading up behind the eye. The onset is rapid over minutes and lasts up to two hours declining as rapidly as it had arisen. It may be so severe as to make it impossible for the sufferer to continue normal activities. Classically it is associated with a stuffy nose and a running red eye. It may happen many times on the same day and is noted for its occurrence at similar times in each day. The sufferer has bouts where the pain occurs over a few weeks with remissions to weeks, months or even years. Between episodes there is total relief from pain. It has associations with migraine — the patient may suffer separate migraine attacks affecting the head and there is often a family history.

Management. Unlike true migraine, the pain is seldom accompanied by nausea, and thus oral medications may be given. Unfortunately medicines taken by mouth are generally too slow in action to prevent the pain developing. Consequently, ordinary analgesics are of limited value, although aspirin and paracetamol compounds do reduce the

pain which has already developed. The specific treatment is ergotamine in a form which is readily and rapidly absorbed. This must be
taken immediately the patient feels that the pain may be developing.
For further information see Chapter 15.

Secondary herpes zoster (shingles)

The virus of herpes zoster produces chickenpox. Secondary herpes
zoster (shingles) generally affects those over 60, but can affect almost
any age. The resulting vesicles and post-herpetic neuralgia affecting
one or two specific peripheral nerves is well known but what is less
recognized is the severe dull pain which occurs in the prodromal
stage, two or three days before the vesicles develop. This pain is
unilateral and dull, starting as a burning sensation which rapidly
progresses to a deep and severe ache. There may by dysaesthesia but
this may not be recognized by the patient because the pain is so
severe. It is at this stage that the patient will present to the dental
practitioner if the second or the third divisions of the trigeminal nerve
are involved. No specific tooth can be implicated, but the patient
may insist upon treatment by extraction and blame the practitioner
for the severe mucosal and cutaneous infection which follows. Where
there is suspicion that herpes zoster may be the cause, the mucosa
and skin in the infected area may be examined for signs of early
inflammation and extraction avoided.

The chronic phase of postherpetic neuralgia is the most distressing
of all the facial pains because it has no cure; patients have been
known to become suicidal. In waking hours, with the patient's mind
occupied, the pain seems not to be intrusive. In the quiet of the
night however the pain becomes dull, insistent and boring, and is
accompanied by a persistent irritation in the affected division of the
nerve. The patient, in looking for relief, may scratch or pick at the
skin to a degree that they draw blood and produce chronic sores.
The skin is usually atrophic.

Management. In the acute phase, treat with analgesics, and prescribe
antibiotics when secondary infection is anticipated (see also Chapter
5, p. 45.). The management of postherpetic neuralgia is unsatisfactory
in that, in the chronic phase, particularly in the elderly, no treatment
is really effective. A combination of tricyclic antidepressants, anticon-
vulsants and local anaesthetic creams to the affected division, may
be of help. For details see Chapter 15.

Cranial arteritis

This is an unusual condition affecting those over 60, females more commonly than males. Although the pain is generally felt on the side of the head behind the eye, it may be felt in the mid or lower face, develops rapidly over a period of days and is constant and increasing during that time. Where it affects the mid or lower face, activity of the masticatory muscles may increase it and rest relieve it. Palpation over prominent arteries such as the superficial temporal, may elicit tenderness. As this is a disease which causes inflammation and occlusion in arteries, characteristically the erythrocyte sedimentation rate (ESR) is found to be raised and treatment is started on suspicion. The patient's medical practitioner should be alerted to the problem immediately because within a matter of days, where the retinal artery is involved, the patient may lose sight in the affected eye. Acute necrosis of facial tissues has been reported.

Management. Refer by telephone to the hospital for medical supervision which generally entails administration of a high dose of systemic steroids.

Tumours

Tumours which develop anywhere along the intracranial or extracranial course of the trigeminal nerve, may cause unilateral dull pain. An acoustic neuroma, causing compression of the trigeminal nerve near the ganglion, produces facial pain and mimics more commonly occurring conditions. As it arises on the eighth cranial nerve, there may be reduced hearing on that side, or symptoms suggesting vestibular involvement. Malignant tumours arising in the postnasal space likewise can mimic other causes of facial pain.

It is important for the clinician to be alert to the possible presence of a tumour whenever the signs and symptoms do not accord with known causes of facial pain. On suspicion, referral to the appropriate specialist is recommended.

III BILATERAL DULL PAIN
Sinusitis

This usually follows a 'cold', and may present as dull unilateral pain over the maxillary sinus, but soon spreads to the other side to become bilateral. Characteristically the pain is worsened by bending down, or jarring the head. It has a dull throbbing character and is often associated with pyrexia. Pressure over the anterior antral wall will cause additional pain. Frequently there is a history of recurrent sinusitis as a result of anatomical abnormalities in the nose such as a deviated septum. The subsequent diagnosis in such persons is then straightforward.

Management. Prescribe antibiotics such as ampicillin (250 mg four times a day for five days), decongestants such as 0.1% Otrivine (which is available without prescription). These usually suffice in the acute stage. Recurrent cases should seek treatment from an otolaryngologist. For details of hospital treatment see Chapter 15.

Atypical facial pain

This is a condition which affects predominantly females and is a diagnosis which should be made only when all other diagnoses have been discarded. Generally affecting young to middle-aged females, it presents as a dull pain which may start unilaterally but generally spreads across the face. The most common area is in the mid-face including the nose, sometimes spreading over the cheeks. The particular features are that it is a dull continuous pain which does not confine itself to known anatomical land-marks, responds poorly to analgesics and seldom interferes with sleep. The patient may describe the pain as severe, yet will be able to carry on a fairly normal life.

Atypical facial pain is associated with depression, particularly where there is anxiety. The pain itself may produce anxiety, the patient fearing a serious condition like cancer, and a vicious circle develops.

Management. After exclusion of genuine pathology, foremost is the requirement of reassurance for the patient. The specific drug therapy required is not available for the dental surgeon, in the British National Formulary. For further formation, refer to Chapter 15.

Atypical Odontalgia

This occurs almost exclusively in young to middle-aged dentally conscious females. Initially it may be confined to one tooth and so much does it mimic pulpitis, that in desperation a dental practitioner may well extirpate the pulp, and ultimately extract the tooth. The characteristics of the pain are dull and continuous, little improved by analgesics — typical of a moderate to severe pulpitis. The offending tooth even may be sensitive percussion. As each tooth is investigated, root filled or extracted, the pain migrates to a further tooth, until the patient and the dental practitioner become equally perplexed, anxious and desperate. Events get increasingly out of hand if the patient is a spouse, dental nurse or mother-in-law!

Management. Primary management begins with referral to a third party, preferably a consultant in oral surgery/oral medicine. After investigation, all dental treatment must be withdrawn, the condition explained to the patient in broad terms, and tricyclic drugs, perhaps with sedation, prescribed as for atypical facial pain. Further dental treatment and investigation should not be started for three months (*see* Chapter 15).

Summary

The diagnosis of facial pain is often difficult, but if the steps are followed as recommended above, most will become straightforward. Of utmost importance is the differentiation between sharp and dull pain, and whether it is unilateral or bilateral.

2: Acute Swellings Related to Dental Tissues

Acute swellings related to dental structures may be divided conveniently into *intra-oral* and *extra-oral* swellings.

I ACUTE INTRA-ORAL SWELLINGS

The most common acute intra-oral swellings are:

1. Acute periapical abscess
2. Acute periodontal abscess
3. Gingival abscess
4. Pericoronitis
5. Haematoma
6. An infected cyst (odontogenic or rarely developmental)
7. Peritonsillar abscess (quinsy)

Bear in mind: swellings at the junction of the hard and soft palate might be tumours of the minor salivary glands, and swellings in the floor of the mouth may arise from the sublingual or submandibular salivary gland. One such swelling in this site is known as a ranula which arises from the sublingual gland. Resist the temptation to incise any of these swellings unless you are sure that they contain pus. Incising a ranula will give no benefit because it will return and may become infected.

Some other common swellings, which perhaps are not defined as acute in the pathological sense but which might well be acute for the patient, are:

- Pyogenic granuloma
- Pregnancy epulis
- Traumatized denture granuloma
- Herniated antral lining through an oro-antral fistula

Methods of investigation

1.   The *dental history* must include:
     (a)   Pain or tenderness prior to the appearance of the swelling
     (b)   The length of time the swelling had been present
     (c)   Preceding dental procedures
     (d)   Signs of bleeding from the swelling.

2.   The *clinical examination* must include:
     (a)   Site
     (b)   Size
     (c)   Colour
     (d)   Consistency—hard, firm, soft, fluctuant.
     (e)   Fixation to the surrounding tissues.
     (f)   Associated lymphadenopathy.

3.   *Special tests* include:
     (a)   *Radiographs.* In dental practice when periapical views are taken it is wise to make two exposures from differing angles. Panoramic radiographs are a useful adjunct but there is a relatively poor definition of detail.
     (b)   *Aspiration.* The aspirant might be:
            (i)   pus from an abscess
            (ii)   air from the maxillary antrum
            (iii) straw coloured fluid from an uninfected cyst
            (iv)   no aspirant from a solid tumour.

Acute periapical abscess (see also Chapter 10, page 88)

This is the consequence of irreversible pulpitis. If the inflammation progresses to an extraoral swelling the site is dependent upon the relationship of the apex of the tooth to the insertions of the orofacial musculature.

Usually the swelling is preceded by bouts of constant, severe pain. The patient is often able to locate the offending tooth because it becomes tender on biting.

Clinical examination reveals a soft, erythematous swelling on the mucosa adjacent to the root of the offending tooth. The swelling sometimes points or discharges and sometimes pus may be extruded from the gingival crevice if pressure is applied over it. The affected tooth will be painful to percussion.

A swelling presenting in the palate often arises from the apical area of an upper lateral incisor, or from the palatal root of a two rooted upper premolar or upper molar.

Radiological examination usually reveals an area of apical radio-lucency by the time a swelling is clinically evident. *Always* take two periapical radiographs taken from differing angles.

Special tests: the offending tooth will not respond to hot or cold stimuli nor to the electric pulp tester.

Management will depend on:

- The condition of the involved tooth
- The degree of bone destruction as seen on the radiograph
- The importance of the tooth as an abutment for a fixed or removable prosthesis
- Whether the tooth is a primary or secondary tooth
- The overall state of the mouth, and the attitude (wishes?) of the patient.

Management

1. Establish drainage preferably via the root canal. Instruct the patient to use hot mouthwashes hourly.
2. Make a small incision at the most fluctuant part of the swelling to elicit drainage when the swelling is very large and drainage via the root canal is not adequate. This procedure may be carried out by placing a topical anaesthetic paste or spraying ethyl chloride over the site of the intended incision and 'stabbing' the swelling with a No. 11. scalpel blade.
3. Prescribe antibiotics when drainage has been unproductive or if there is a pyrexia, and painful and increasing lymphadenopathy.
4. Extract the offending tooth after the acute infection has subsided, or immediately under a general anaesthetic.

Bear in mind: if a primary tooth, is involved give consideration to the presence, position and state of development of the permanent successor before deciding to extract, (*see* Chapter 3).

Acute periodontal abscess

The most common complaint is the sudden onset of a deep boring pain in a tooth on which the patient has been tending to clench. Pressure of the occlusion will relieve discomfort in the early stages of the lesion. In the later stages, the discomfort may be accompanied by a 'nasty taste' and spontaneous bleeding. The adjacent tooth is tender to bite on and is sometimes slightly mobile. In the early stages there may be no discharge but later pus may be extruded from the gingival crevice or from a sinus in the mucosa overlying the affected root. This makes the differentiation from a periapical abscess more difficult; pulp tests are often misleading.

The overlying gingival tissues are red, tender and swollen. Once there is a discharge of pus into the mouth or into the soft tissues there is an immediate abatement of severe pain.

Management. Depends on the stage at which the patient presents.

1. In the early stage treat with antibiotics (penicillin 250 mg four times a day for five days, metronidazole 200 mg three times a day hourly for five days or erythromycin 250 mg four times a day for five days).
2. Instruct the patient to use hot mouthwashes hourly.
3. Adjust the opposing tooth so that there is no occlusal contact.
4. Ensure that the patient returns for further treatment after the acute phase has subsided.
5. Establish drainage if the abscess is fluctuant. Use a topical anaesthetic paste or an ethyl chloride spray prior to incising through the point of maximum fluctuation using a No 11 or 15 blade. If local anaesthesia is used, always inject well away from the infected area preferably using block anaesthesia. Instruct the patient to use hot mouthwashes hourly. Antibiotics may not be required if drainage is adequate.
6. A localized abscess may progress to a cellulitis. When spread into the soft tissues is suspected, intramuscular antibiotics (*see* Appendix) must be administered.
7. Initiate endodontic therapy after the acute phase has subsided if a combined perio-endo lesion is suspected.
8. Extract if there has been a great amount of destruction of the supporting tissues of the tooth.

Gingival abscess

This is usually associated with physical damage to the gingival tissues as sometimes happens with a woodstick. It appears as a localized red swelling. The adjacent teeth may be tender to bite on.

Management. Remove the cause if still present and establish drainage. Instruct patient to use hot mouthwashes hourly.

Periocoronitis

This is an infection arising beneath a gum flap around the crown of a partially erupted tooth. It most commonly affects the lower third molar, rarely the upper third molar. The patient complains of constant pain, often severe and radiating from the offending tooth.

The clinical signs are an erythematous flap of tissue partially covering the offending tooth from which pus may flow if it is lifted with a blunt probe. This tissue and part of the adjacent cheek may be ulcerated. Other signs and symptoms may include:

- Trismus
- Foetor oris
- Facial swelling over the angle of the mandible.
- Lymphadenitis
- Pyrexia

Bear in mind: a migrating abscess may occur from the site of the pericoronitis and appear as a pointing abscess on the buccal aspect of the lower second or even first molar.

Management.

1. *Local*: irrigate beneath the gum flap. This is sometimes exceedingly difficult if trismus is severe. Apply trichloracetic acid *with extreme care* beneath the gum flap: always neutralize with glycerine before discharging the patient.

If indicated, adjust the occlusal surface of the upper third molar so that the gum flap is no longer traumatized, or extract the upper third molar if the treatment plan allows. Removal of the gum flap is rarely effective in the long-term and should not be attempted in the acute phase.

2. *General*: instruct patient to use hot mouthwashes hourly. Prescribe metronidazole 200 mg three times a day for five days, or penicillin V 250 mg four times a day for five days. Review at a later date for removal of the lower third molar.

Haematoma

This is usually associated with trauma. The presence of a sub-lingual haematoma is strongly suggestive of a fracture of the body of the mandible.

Bear in mind: patients on anticoagulant medication may develop a haematoma rapidly at sites of periodontal infection and pericoronitis.

Perforation of a root

This is often associated with a recent attempt at endodontic therapy, a post crown preparation or the placement of a pin retained core.

Clinical examination reveals a slight erythematous swelling on the soft tissue located over the central third of a root (rather than over the apex). Differential diagnosis must include an early periodontal abscess.

Management.

1. Raise a flap and seal the perforation with amalgam when the perforation is on the buccal aspect of the root and the access is straightforward (not necessarily the case on all premolars and molars). The patient must return for a post operative check at 5–7 days.
2. Advise extraction if the perforation is on the palatal aspect the chances of a good repair are slight.

Bear in mind: following the repair of the perforation, usually the tooth will have to be re-restored. If the amount of root remaining is not sufficient to retain a replacement post, extract the root.

3. Remove the restoration and the offending pins if they have been found to have penetrated the pulp chamber or the periodontal membrane space. Properly restore the tooth. If these pins have penetrated the pulp chamber, commence endodontic therapy.

Peritonsillar abscess (quinsy)

Infection around the tonsillar area may involve both pillars of the fauces and produce a swelling in the soft palate. The condition mimics a pericoronitis associated with an upper third molar. The patient complains of a severe soreness in the throat, difficulty in swallowing and present usually with trismus.

Management. Refer to the department of otolaryngology at the nearest hospital. There is a problem in these cases for the anaesthetist because the trismus demands that a nasal tube has to be used for the intubation. There is the associated danger that the abscess can be ruptured and the pus drain directly down into the area of the larynx.

II ACUTE EXTRAORAL SWELLINGS

In practice almost all acute discrete swellings in the orofacial tissues are due to infection, and most of these arise from the teeth and associated supporting tissues. Look for:

- Tenderness
- Redness
- Fluctuation: this may be difficult to elicit in the orofacial tissues, especially where there is much associated oedema. Palpate bimanually over the swelling, feel over the alveolus intraorally and extraorally. Locate the point of maximum fluctuation if possible.
- Fixation: try to move the swelling across the underlying structures, and try to move the skin over the swelling. If the swelling is tethered to the skin, it indicates that the inflammatory process is becoming superficial and may point soon.
- Trismus: this indicates that the inflammatory process has progressed to involve the pterygo-masseteric sling. It may mean that there is pus beneath one or both these muscles. This requires urgent treatment.

Bear in mind:

- ▲ A non-tender, nonfluctuant swelling may be a tumour.
- ▲ A non-fluctuant, red painful swelling may represent an aggressive malignant tumour about to rupture the skin.
- ▲ Acute inflammatory swellings may arise in pre-existing pathological conditions.

Differential diagnosis

Where there are acute inflammatory swellings in the orofacial tissues, *first exclude a dental cause* and then consider:

The lymph nodes

- Bacterial infections may be secondary to infections in the dental tissues but consider also the primary infections in the nasopharynx, the tonsils, the ears, the scalp and other parts of the face.

     In the under-twelves, primary staphylococcal infection of the cervical lymph nodes is quite common. In the over-twelves, enlarged cervical lymph nodes may be 'reactive' to acne.
- Viral infections, particularly measles and glandular fever. The latter may start with unilateral lymph node swelling. Measles usually causes multiple small nodes, particularly in the posterior cervical group.

- The reticuloses. Usually the swellings are neither tender nor acute.

The skin. Infections in the hair follicles (boils), and in pre-existing sebaceous cysts.

The salivary glands. The sumandibular salivary gland is most prone to infection due to its great propensity to have stones blocking its duct. Initially the swelling may be non-infective with a history of swelling at the thought, sight or taste of food. Ascending infection may supervene. Bimanual palpation will elicit a swollen, tender and possibly fluctuant submandibular salivary gland. This is difficult to differentiate from an infected lymph node. Inspect the floor of the mouth. Any redness or swelling in the path of the sumandibular duct suggests that the swelling is arising in the submandibular salivary gland.

The parotid gland becomes infected less frequently than the sumandibular gland and produces a characteristic swelling at the front of the ear. Always inspect for the presence of pus at the parotid papilla, milking across the masseter if necessary. Usually suppurative parotitis is restricted to the dehydrated patient and those debilitated by systemic disease.

Infectious fevers. Mumps is the most common infectious fever to affect the parotid glands. It may affect the submandibular salivary glands too. Swelling of the parenchyma of the parotid gland *may be* caused by glandular fever, and other viruses.

Haematoma. This is almost always associated with a history of trauma. Haematoma may become encysted, particularly in the elderly: these haematoma are subject to infection. *Where there is no convincing history of trauma sufficient to cause the evident haematoma, bear in mind*:

▲ Pathological fracture — fracture through a mandible weakened by pre-existing pathology.
▲ Severe blood dyscrasia
▲ The patient may be taking steroids
▲ The patient may be taking anticoagulant drugs
▲ The patient is elderly, with atrophic tissue
▲ Bleeding into a pre-existing tumour – rare

Tumours. Acute presentation is due usually to infection in an ulcerated tumour or bleeding from an eroded vessel.

Mucous extravasation cysts. The most common site is the lower lip. They occur in the young to middle aged, and are thought to be the result of trauma damaging the duct of a small mucous gland. The gland secretes into the soft tissues of the lip. A small blue fluctuant swelling is the result.

Generalized swelling of the facial tissues. This may be caused by angio-oedema and an allergic response to, for example, bee stings and insect bites.

Surgical emphysema. This arises as a result of:

▲ Accidental inflation of the soft tissues from the exhaust of an airotor
▲ Using a 'three-in-one' syringe to dry out the contents of a root canal
▲ The patient blowing the nose after a successful repair of an oroantral fistula
▲ Injuries to the neck causing air from the oesophagus or trachea to enter the soft tissues. This is extremely dangerous and requires urgent hospital attention.

Special investigations for acute extraoral swellings:

1. Always take the patient's temperature
2. Take radiographs to exclude tooth and bone pathology — extra-oral films such as an orthopantomagram or lateral oblique radiographs may be required
3. Needle aspiration in some cases.

Management. Most cases of acute extra-oral swelling will require referral to a Department of Oral Surgery for further investigation and treatment. *Where there is pyrexia refer to hospital immediately, telephoning the on-call team first.*

If you are satisfied that you can handle the infection yourself,

1. Prescribe antibiotics. Penicillin V 500 mg four times a day for five days, Ampicillin 250 mg four times a day for five days or metronidazole 200 mg three times a days for five days. For infections you believe to be more severe, amoxycillin 250 mg three times a day for five days together with metronidazole 200 mg three times a day.
2. Encourage good fluid intake.
3. The patient should be off work.
4. If the patient is worse after 24 hours or no better at 48 hours, *double the dose of antibiotics.*
5. If the patient remains no better after a further 48 hours, *refer to hospital by telephone.*

TOPOGRAPHICAL LISTING OF SWELLINGS OF THE OROFACIAL TISSUES

Angle of the mandible

- Abscesses on lower molar teeth
- Pericoronitis around an erupting wisdom tooth
- Submasseteric abscess

Swellings at the side of the neck

- Extensions downwards from abscesses above
- Primary bacterial infections of the lymph nodes (particulary children 12 and under)
- Primary infection of the lymph nodes from systemic viral infections
- Secondary infection of lymph nodes (from teeth as above, tonsils, possibly ear, scalp or skin)
- Infections of the submandibular salivary gland — usually bacterial, very rarely viral
- Submandibular salivary gland with a blocked duct
- Infected branchial cyst, (rare)
- Actinomycosis
- Emphysema from a damaged trachea or oesophagus.

Body of the mandible

- Infections arising from the lower premolars and molars
- Infection of the masseteric lymph node. Occurs particularly following the removal of an impacted lower third molar where there is a mild 'dry socket'. Any adjacent intra-oral infection may cause it.

Anterior mandible and chin

- Infections arising from lower canines
- Mucous extravasation cyst from the floor of the mouth — a ranula (this may become infected)
- Reactive lymph nodes — from acne.

Generalized swelling of the neck

- Cellulitis (Ludwig's angina) — infection spreading from any of the above, usually caused by a mixed infection of aerobes and

anaerobes. It is particularly dangerous because it advances rapidly and may cause oedema of the glottis.
- Surgical emphysema from the exhaust from an airotor into the soft tissues of the root canal of lower teeth.

Periorbital

- Infections arising from upper anterior teeth particularly the canine
- Infections in the eyes
- Dacrocystitis and infections of the lachrymal apparatus
- Unusually, sinusitis
- Surgical emphysema from nose blowing after a repair of an oro-antral fistula, or from the exhaust from an airotor.

Alae of the nose and upper lip

- Infections arising from upper incisor teeth
- Surgical emphysema from the exhaust of an airotor used on upper anterior teeth or the root canals of upper anterior teeth
- Allergic effects — usually in association with the lower lip.

Lower lip

- Infections involving the lower anterior teeth
- Mucous extravasation cyst
- Infected lacerations — the lower lip is prone to damage from the upper incisor teeth as a consequence of falls etc
- Allergic effects — usually in association with the upper lip (see also Chapter 5, p. 52).

Cheeks

- Infections arising from the upper premolar and molar teeth
- Sinusitis (rarely)
- The skin — infected hair follicles, sebaceous cysts.

3:   Trauma

In this section the management of *trauma* will be outlined in relation
to:

- Trauma to the soft tissues
- Trauma to the primary dentition
- Trauma to the permanent teeth: anterior and posterior

For fractures of the facial skeleton see Chapter 17, p. 147. For trauma
to the temperomandibular joint see Chapter 15, page 121.

GENERAL CONSIDERATIONS

It may be expected that most patients receiving trauma to the facial
tissues and the facial skeleton will present to the accident and
emergency department of the local hospital. However this is by no
means always the case and there are occasions when minor trauma
is referred back to the general dental practitioner or it has remained
unrecognized by the casualty officer on duty. Fractures of the facial
bones and most facial lacerations will require management in hospital,
but many of the more minor injuries may be dealt with satisfactorily
in a dental practice.

No matter how minor the injury, *take careful history* of the injury
itself, and a medical history of the patient. The important points of
each are:

History of the injury

1. The circumstances — was it accidental, was it an assault, what
   happened before and after the injury, what sort of first aid
   treatment was carried out?
2. Did the patient lose consciousness — could the consequences of
   head injury develop.
3. What instrument caused the injury which you are examining? Is
   it a clean injury or might there be a foreign body in it? Might it
   be a deep penetrating injury with a small external hole?

4. Might the injury have been caused by a missile which may still remain in the tissues.
5. How long ago was the injury caused?
6. Has there been much blood loss?

Important points in the medical history

1. Is there a bleeding diathesis?
2. Is there intercurrent disease which could lead to decreased resistance to infection?
3. Is the patient an epileptic? If the injury was as the result of a fall, might it have been caused by a momentary loss of consciousness — sometimes known as a drop attack?
4. What medication is the patient taking?

If you are satisfied from the above history that the injury is uncomplicated, and you feel competent to treat it, consider the following.

I SOFT TISSUES

In a dental practice the treatment of lacerations should be restricted to small fresh wounds generally involving the oral tissues only.

1. Consider what may have caused the injury
2. Inspect the wound carefully and assess whether the wound correlates well with the history
3. Take a soft tissue radiograph if it is felt that a foreign body might be present. Where there are fractured teeth, there is always a possibility that fragments of the teeth remain in the wound — particulary the lower lip. Intra-oral films are invaluable in revealing foreign bodies when placed close to the wound, using a reduced exposure and/or increased tube-film distance.
4. Inject local anaesthetic solution — it is more comfortable for the patient, if the needle is inserted through the laceration. Local anaesthetic preparations containing adrenaline are ideal. Infiltrate for up to 2 cms all round the laceration.
5. Explore the wound under a good light to assess the structures that might have been damaged in the depths of the wound. Explore with a probe for foreign material. Be prepared to tie off or cauterize vessels which may bleed.
6. If there is dehiscence in the muscle, for example in the orbicularis oris, suture this with absorbable material such as 3–0 catgut. Suture the mucosa. Materials for such suturing are a matter of personal preference with non-absorbable silk, artificial fibre and absorbable catgut all being used.
7. Tears in the depths of the sulcus such as the 'degloving' injury over a bony prominence of the chin are best left unsutured. External support of the lip with elastoplast may be helpful. This is achieved best by 1 inch stretchable elastoplast; cut a piece about 12 inches (25 cm) long, stick one end across the cheek just above the lower border of the mandible, stretch the next portion horizontally beneath the lower lip and with tension just above the chin point. Fix the remainder across the opposite cheek, to match the first side.
8. Lacerations of the tongue seldom need suturing, unless longer than 1.5 cm. If bleeding persists from the deeper tissues, this must be controlled before the mucosa is sutured.

Bear in mind: ducts of the salivary gland, motor and sensory nerves may have been involved.

Lacerations of the tongue and the floor of the mouth may lead to considerable swelling of the tongue. If in doubt refer to the hospital.

II TRAUMA TO THE PRIMARY DENTITION

Most injuries to primary teeth are a result of vertical forces and the maxillary anterior teeth are most commonly involved.

The injury is usually reported by telephone by the parent or a guardian (school teacher). Obtain a brief history of the accident and attempt to reassure the caller who is usually very anxious. Consideration must always be given to the permanent successor.

Make an immediate appointment at the practice or at the local hospital. The history should indicate if the child has sustained injuries other than to the dental tissues which might require attention at the Accident and Emergency department of the local hospital.

The patient may present with:

1. No apparent clinical or radiographical problems. The parents must be warned of the possibility of pain, swelling or discolouration of the tooth.
2. *Mobility*: mobility of 0–2 mm does not require stabilization. Extract the tooth if mobility is excessive as a result of alveolar bone fracture.
3. *Displacement*: a tooth which is displaced palatally can be left if it does not interfere with the occlusion.

Extract the tooth if there is a labial displacement of the crown thereby reducing the possibility of damage to the permanent successor, or if the tooth is so mobile that there is a danger of the child inhaling it.

4. *Intrusion*: the result of intrusion can be that the entire clinical crown may not be visible in the mouth. The presence of the tooth must be confirmed by taking a radiograph. The patient is not usually in any discomfort and the management is reassurance. The teeth usually reposition themselves over a period of a few weeks.
5. *Avulsion*: an avulsed primary maxillary incisor need not be re-implanted. Loss of the residual space is unlikely.
6. *Discolouration*: varying degrees of discolouration can arise over a few days in traumatized primary teeth, weeks or even months after the injury has occurred. This eventuality may be more a problem for the patient, or even the parent, than for the practitioner. It requires no management other than reassurance unless there is a suspicion of periapical infection. In such a case endodontic therapy must be instituted or the primary tooth extracted to avoid damage to the developing permanent successor.

7. *Fracture*: the fracture of the crown or a root of a primary anterior
    tooth rarely occurs although it may happen as a result of carious
    breakdown of the crown. The management depends on the age
    of the patient and the degree of coronal destruction and pulpal
    involvement. It can range from smoothing the sharp edges of the
    fractured crown, endodontic intervention or extraction.

III TRAUMA TO THE PERMANENT DENTITION

This can be divided into:

- Partially avulsed teeth
- Completely avulsed teeth
- Anterior tooth crown fracture
- Anterior tooth root fracture
- Posterior tooth crown fracture
- Posterior tooth root fracture

General considerations

1. The *history* must include the time and manner in which the trauma was inflicted.
2. *Clinical examination* must not only be related to the traumatized tooth or teeth. Soft tissue lacerations must be palpated or probed for the presence of tooth tissue or other foreign bodies as described on page 148.
3. Adjacent and *opposing* teeth must be examined for evidence of involvement. In those situations where anterior teeth are fractured *always* examine posterior teeth which might also be involved.
4. *Radiological examination* must be made of all teeth suspected to have been involved. Two exposures at differing angles have to be available for each of the teeth.
5. Always warn the patient (or the parent) that in future the pulps of the involved teeth might become necrosed.
6. Ensure that the records are completed immediately and contain all details of the incident and the treatment carried out. Such information may have to be produced if legal proceedings are preferred.

Partially avulsed tooth

This requires immediate treatment to prevent root resorption. The tooth may be partially displaced or intruded.

Management. Reposition the tooth as quickly as possible after the injury. If there is extreme mobility, splint with an acid etch/wire splint. Pulp test the tooth at this stage with an electric pulp tester if only to create a baseline for further reference.

If the tooth is discoloured or is symptomatic, commence endodontic therapy.

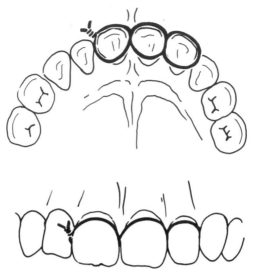

Fig. 3.1 Where a tooth is subluxed, a simple figure-of-eight is an effective splint

Completely avulsed tooth

The basic premise is to keep the socket clean and replant the tooth as quickly as possible. Therefore instructions given on the telephone are very important; tell the patient to wash the tooth under running water, attempt to re-implant it and come immediately to the practice.

If the tooth cannot be re-implanted at the place where the accident occurred, instruct the patient to transport the tooth to the practice in a plastic bag filled with saline (a teaspoon of salt in a glass of warm water) — if possible!. An adult patient may be advised to keep the avulsed tooth in the mouth under the tongue or in the buccal vestibule so that it is constantly bathed in saliva.

On arrival at the practice:

1. Check the re-implanted tooth for position, assess the degree of mobility and splint using acid etch/wire mesh/composite resin splint if necessary. Take a radiograph to see if the alveolus or an adjacent root has been fractured during the incident.

2. Prior to re-implantation do not touch the root of the avulsed tooth or attempt to scrape off debris. Wash the tooth under running tap water holding it in tweezers by the coronal portion only.
3. Gently irrigate the socket making every effort not to touch the walls. It may be necessary sometimes to make a small relieving hole through the buccal plate, level with the apex of the socket to allow for more precise positioning of the tooth.
4. If the tooth has been out of the mouth longer than two hours, endodontic therapy is indicated prior to re-implantation.
5. Once repositioned, stabilize the tooth with acid etch/wire splint for four weeks.
6. Warn the patient or the parent of the dangers of pulp necrosis, root resorption or ankylosis all which may occur in the future.

Anterior tooth crown fracture

1. *Fracture only in enamel*: usually this requires smoothing of the enamel edges only but the traumatized teeth are very prone to pulp necrosis at a later date. Take radiographs and pulp test the tooth making a note of the degree of response.
2. *Fracture involving dentine but no exposure*: protect any exposed dentine with calcium hydroxide and a cover of composite material. Take radiographs and pulp test the tooth making a note of the degree of response.
3. *Fracture involving pulp in tooth with open apex*: carry out a pulpotomy; this allows for completion of apical development. Seal calcium hydroxide into the canal for four months. Orthograde endodontics may be carried out at a later date.
4. *Fracture involving pulp of the tooth with closed apex*: carry out routine endodontic therapy. The chances of success with pulp capping are reduced because of contamination of the exposure with saliva etc.

Anterior tooth root fracture

1. *Horizontal fracture in the apical third of a root*: once the diagnosis has been confirmed clinically and radiographically no treatment is required. The patient is told to attend periodically for pulp testing and follow up radiographs.

2. *Horizontal fracture in the middle third of a root*: treat much as an apical third root fracture except that the tooth will have to be splinted with acid etch/wire splint.
3. *Vertical and oblique fractures*: Abscess formation may be the first clinical sign of vertical root fracture and it may occur equally on vital and non-vital roots. Pain on chewing which steadily gets worse is common. Radiographs may only show a thickened periodontal membrane and probing may reveal a pocket in the affected area. A flap procedure may be required to confirm the diagnosis.

If an oblique fracture of a root finishes below the level of the crestal bone, it is very difficult to restore the remainder of the root. It may be possible to extrude the root a little using an orthodontic appliance.

Always ensure that there is sufficient root remaining to permit the retention of a subsequent restoration.

Extract a root if it is fractured vertically.

Posterior tooth – crown fracture

This happens often as a sequel to a cracked tooth. If dentine is exposed, the glass ionomer cements provide an excellent protective provisional repair material. If time and circumstance permit place a definitive restoration using a small pin for increased retention if required.

Posterior tooth – root fracture

The management of these fractures is similar to that in anterior tooth root fracture except that each root has to be considered separately.

Management. Extract the tooth if the fracture line runs mesio-distally through the crown of the tooth.

If the fracture line passes bucco-lingually through the furcation area and between the roots it may be possible to remove the isolated root. A restoration may be made which is supported by the remaining roots after endodontic therapy. When a fracture occurs between the roots of a two rooted upper premolar, the tooth is unsaveable.

4: Haemorrhage From The Mouth

Haemorrhage from the mouth is commonly the result of:

- Tooth extraction — this may be primary, reactionary, or secondary (see later).
- Accidental laceration of soft tissue.

It may be caused by:

- Gingival bleeding as a result of periodontal conditions (Chapter 11).
- Bleeding from telangiectasis or haemangioma.
- A broken denture or appliance.
- A ruptured abscess — spontaneous rupture discharges pus; blood may follow and resist control, flowing from dilated vessels.
- An eroded vessel in a malignant lesion.

For all haemorrhages in the mouth there *may be* general factors and there *will be* local factors.

The following drugs and conditions should be borne in mind

1. *Anticoagulants.* Many patients are taking anticoagulants for a variety of reasons; young women for recurrent deep vein thrombosis, middle aged men following a myocardial infarct or heart valve replacement, old people to avoid a second stroke. Take a good history.
2. *Aspirin* is a mild anticoagulant. Many patients are on regular aspirin dosage to reduce platelet aggregation and avoid thrombosis. This dose is so small as to make no significant difference in bleeding from lesions in the mouth. Large doses for example given to patients with rheumatoid arthritis, could have a significant effect to extend the clotting time. Patients in pain may take doses well in excess of the recommended dose, and be unaware of the content of proprietary analgesic preparations. Take a good history.
3. *Haemophilia or Christmas Disease.* When these conditions are severe enough to cause spontaneous bleeding from the mouth, it is highly likely the patient will already know that they suffer from

the disease. Mild forms however, may be unmasked by tooth extraction and generally present as reactionary haemorrhage.

4. *Platelet disorders.* Leukaemia and thrombocytopenia may cause spontaneous bleeding from the gingivae or be an embarrassment following tooth extraction. Generally, however, there are other signs of the disease and it is unlikely that the patient will present to a dental practitioner without the diagnosis already having been made. A continous ooze from the gingivae however, should be considered suspicious and further surgery avoided until the medical condition has been investigated.

5. *Patients become very alarmed at haemorrhage from the mouth.* This itself can raise the blood pressure and this may contribute to the bleeding. Additionally, anxiety raises fibrinolysin levels. More importantly, repeated mouth washing, interference from the tongue or meddling by the patient or a relative with a bleeding tooth socket, can maintain bleeding indefinitely.

Tooth extraction (post extraction haemorrhage)

This may be:

- Primary — occurring at the time of surgery
- Reactionary — occurring when the arterioles dilate as the effects of the adrenaline in the local anaesthetic wear off
- Secondary — as a result of infection. Only virulent infections bleed within 24 hours after tooth extraction. Previously uninfected sockets usually do not bleed for about 48 hours.

There may be other local factors:

- Pre-existing gingival inflammation causing an increased blood supply in dilated vessels
- Tears in the gingivae. A torn vessel is unable to constrict and retract
- Fractured alveolar process (tuberosity). In part this is due to a tear in a vessel, and in part due to mobility across the fracture
- Fractured jaw (rare)
- Unrecognized tumour (very rare)

Management. Local measures are the basis of all treatment of post-extraction haemorrhage even though there may be a systemic underlying cause. Every attempt must be made to make the conditions ideal locally for clotting to take place. Careful techniques should have been used to remove the tooth, but even with the best of intentions gingival laceration can occur.

Aspirator tip   Gillies toothed dissecting forceps
            Scalpel handle   Kilner cheek retractor

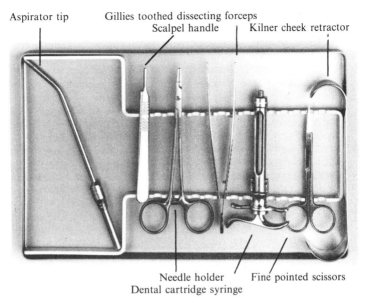

Needle holder   Fine pointed scissors
Dental cartridge syringe

Fig. 4.1   A suturing set

It is essential to react calmly and with confidence, and to take charge of the situation. Generally it is best to separate the patient from a relative or friend. It is important to sit the patient in an upright chair under a good light with a competent person to assist. An aspirator must be available, together with all the necessary instrumentation (for example, a mirror, a small aspirator tip, toothed dissecting forceps, tissue scissors, needle holders, and strong suture material).

1. Inspect the wound — give the patient a mouthwash and remove all the clot in the area of the bleeding using an aspirator.
2. Place a moistened pack over the wound and get the patient to apply pressure by closing the mouth. The pack must be made of woven material and folded to make its bulk no bigger than twice the size of the tooth that has been removed, so that it can exert pressure on the gingival margins. Insert it carefully over the socket and, where appropriate, instruct the patient to bite for 20 minutes without further inspection. Should bleeding still occur

the pack will require repositioning. If bleeding continues, repeat. If bleeding still continues progress to:

3.   Infiltrate around the socket with local anaesthetic containing adrenaline, and wait for two to three minutes. Assistance now becomes necessary. Remove any redundant clot and inspect the wound edges. If the bleeding is from tears or incisions, excise the edges of the wound which are mobile or whose blood supply is in doubt (cyanotic and with a narrow pedicle). Suture deeply into the tissue across any tears or incisions from which the bleeding seems to originate, and tie tightly to compress the tissue.

    Draw the mucosa across the socket using a horizontal mattress suture whenever possible tying the suture tightly until the gingival tissue blanches. Place a pack over the socket, instruct the patient to apply pressure for five minutes and inspect the wound. Once more, if the bleeding is not controlled progress to:

4.   Pack the socket. Whether the local analgesic is still effective or not, infiltrate local anaesthetic solution containing adrenaline around the edges of the wound once more. Remove the mattress suture and replace it, but do not tie. A helpful manoeuvre is to hook the suture material traversing the socket back over the adjacent teeth to leave the socket clear for packing, *see* Fig. 4.2. The pack can be of absorbable or non-absorbable material of a consistency which can be compressed into the wound, for example absorbable Surgicel or non-absorbable ribbon gauze soaked in Whitehead's varnish. Do not use absorbable sponge. Disengage the transversing threads of the mattress suture from the adjacent teeth and lay over the pack. Tie the suture.

Only rarely does this not succeed. If the mucosa is a very badly torn, perhaps with deficiencies over the edge of the socket, do as above but place the sutures further away from the socket and lay Surgicel over the socket in two to three layers. This is stabilized by the transverse strands of the suture.

Rarely if a bleeding point is seen, oversew with purse-string or figure-of-eight suture.

When stage (4) is approached, consider sedating the patient. In the dental surgery, diazepam 5–10 mg or temazepam 10 mg should be adequate, although a very nervous patient may require up to three times the dose. Diazepam may be given intramuscularly or intravenously 5–10 mg provided that the patient does not have upper airway disease. An alternative drug is Midazolam 5–10 mg. All patients who have had sedation must be accompanied, and must not drive or use machinery, even kitchen equipment, for 24 hours.

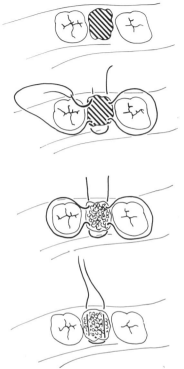

Fig. 4.2 Surgicel sutured into a persistently bleeding socket. Note that the suture is placed before the Surgicel is inserted and is looped over the adjacent teeth. This avoids the difficulties normally encountered if the needle is passed through the mucosa after the Surgicel is placed in the socket

Purpura and Telangiectasia
See Chapter 5, p. 49.

Haemorrhage following periodontal therapy
See Chapter 11, p. 98.

Accidental injury
See Chapter 14.

5: Emergencies Involving The Oral Mucous Membranes

I ULCERATIONS

Ulcers may be traumatic, malignant, idiopathic, or the end-point of bullous, viral and atrophic oral lesions.

Traumatic ulcer

Traumatic ulcers may occur anywhere in the mouth and the source of the trauma is usually evident; for example, the ulcer at the periphery of an over-extended denture, or the ulcer on the side of the tongue adjacent to a recently fractured tooth. Patients may present however after weeks or months of minor discomfort when the features may be alarmingly similar to that of a carcinoma with a hard, raised, everted edge and an indurated base. Local lymph nodes may be enlarged and tender. The enlarged non-tender lymph node should awaken the suspicion of malignancy, particularly if it is hard and irregular in shape.

Management. Remove any obvious cause of the trauma and see the patient one week later. At this stage, if the base of the ulcer is healed and the periphery is less inflamed and less indurated, the diagnosis is confirmed but it is expedient to see the patient again within a further week. If the base of the ulcer remains and the inflammation persists, refer to hospital immediately with an urgent letter or telephone call.

Stomatitis artefacta

This is a curious condition where the patient deliberately damages the oral mucosa by the use of a finger nail or other sharp object but will not necessarily admit to it. Such ulcers have all the features of trauma, but the sources of the trauma is not immediately evident. The commonest sites are in the upper labial mucosa where a finger

40

nail is used, or on the hard or soft palate when an instrument is used. The patients are usually young females with psychiatric disturbance but occasionally it is seen in the older patient with post-herpetic neuralgia, in an area of diminished sensation.

Management. The diagnosis is often difficult to confirm, particularly in those with minor psychiatric disturbance. Counselling may be sufficient. To establish the diagnosis, particularly where the patient denies self trauma, it is helpful to cover the affected area where possible with a temporary splint. A vacuum formed appliance is ideal and it may be necessary to cement it into position for a few days to establish the diagnosis. Referral to a psychiatrist may be necessary. This should be discussed with the patient's Medical Practitioner.

Malignant ulcer

A malignant ulcer may present as described above, with clinical features of a chronic traumatic ulcer, or first as a raised plaque or desquamative lesion within an area of leucoplakia. It may present at the outset within apparently normal mucosa and may arise in the mucous membrane itself or from underlying structures. The ulcer has raised everted edges arising out of a firm indurated base. The most common sites for oral malignancy are in the lower part of the mouth — the lateral border of the tongue, the floor of the mouth, the lower alveolus and the lower lip.

If cervical lymph nodes are detected, and are non-tender and irregular in shape, refer to hospital immediately.

Management. If the ulcer is less than 5 mm in diameter and associated with possible trauma, treat as for a simple traumatic ulcer as described above, and review in a week. If it is larger than 5 mm in diameter refer by urgent letter or a telephone call to hospital for definitive investigation and management.

Recurrent ulceration

Up to 20% of the population suffer aphthous ulceration from time to time, but chronic sufferers often have a family history. Minor trauma to the mucous membrane acts as a trigger. There are three main presentations:

- minor recurrent aphthous ulceration
- major recurrent aphthous ulceration
- stomatitis herpetiformis

Minor recurrent aphthous ulceration is the most common. A crop of six to eight ulcers may be present at any one time, each up to 5 mm, in diameter and lasting seven to ten days. In major recurrent aphthous ulceration, the ulcers are larger, up to a centimetre or more in diameter. Each lasts six to twelve weeks and, unlike minor aphthous ulceration, healing generally is followed by scarring. Scars elsewhere in the mouth may serve as a clue to the diagnosis. Stomatitis herpetiformis is the name given to the condition where multiple small ulcers develop in the mouth, often coalescing into large irregular ulcers. They seldom last more than ten days. All these ulcerations tend to occur predominantly in non-keratinised oral epithelium and in bouts. Some patients with minor aphthous ulceration may seldom be free of symptoms. It is the severe and painful episode which might present as an emergency.

Management. There is no prevention and no cure for this condition. Healing of the ulcers may be assisted by:

1. Tetracycline mouth washes. Break a 250 mg capsule into 10 ml of warm water. Use as a mouth rinse four times a day without swallowing it. This can assist in healing ulcers which have become secondarily infected. Some practitioners prefer a combination mouth wash of Tetracyline and Nystatin (Mysteclin).
2. Chlorhexidine mouthwashes, and miconazole oral gel. These preparations are helpful in reducing secondary infection, used four times per day.
3. Topical steroids — hydrocortisone pellets 2.5 mg. Hold in the mouth as close as possible to the ulcers; 0.1% triamcinolone acetonide in oral adhesive base (Orabase) may be applied directly to the ulcers. This is practical only on relatively immobile mucosa.
4. Systemic steroids. Large areas of ulceration are extremely painful and make it difficult for the patient to take food and fluid. In these circumstances, a short course of systemic steroids is indicated. Prescribe prednisolone in divided doses, starting at 60 mg per day and reducing to nil within ten days. Systemic steroids may be dangerous and should only be prescribed under the direction of a physician.

Bear in mind: middle aged patients presenting for the first time with recurrent aphthous ulceration, may have malabsorption syndrome; thus a careful history should be taken followed by appropriate investigation if malabsorption is suspected (weight loss and frequent pale offensive stools — *see* also Chapter 19).

A few patients with ulcers identical with minor aphthous ulceration, will have Behçet's syndrome. Oral lesions may be accompanied by ulcers on the genitalia and conjunctiva.

Acute necrotising ulcerative gingivitis (Vincent's infection)

The ulceration in this condition is characteristic. It is restricted to the gingival margin causing necrosis particularly of the inter-dental papillae. In the early stages it may be restricted to one quadrant of the mouth but soon spreads to involve the whole mouth. The adjacent gingivae are hyperaemic, bleed easily and are extremely painful. There may be a pyrexia and there will be a characteristic foetid odour. Generally it occurs in those with poor oral hygiene or those debilitated with general disease.

Management. *See* Chapter 11, p. 96

II BULLOUS (BLISTERING) LESIONS

Blistering lesions occur in the mouth either as a result of virus infection or autoimmune disease. Acute burns will not be considered here. When the blisters are small, as in primary Herpes Simplex, they are known as vesicles, and when they are large, they are known as bullae.

Herpes simplex

70–90% of the population are carriers of the virus of herpes simplex. Once the virus is introduced to a susceptible host, usually a child without antibodies to it, an acute gingivo-stomatitis follows. Once the acute infection is over, approximately 1% will suffer recurrent or secondary herpetic lesions.

1. Primary herpetic gingivo-stomatitis

This condition affects children and young adults and manifests as a fever, sore throat and cervical lymphadenopathy. Within days the mouth becomes painful with gingival and then general oral inflammation. Fluid filled vesicles develop which rupture to form shallow, ragged and painful ulcers. Where the vesicles coalesce, the ulcers may reach up to 1 cm in size. Spontaneous resolution occurs within seven to fourteen days.

Management. The herpetic infection cannot be aborted and thus treatment is directed to an early recovery and avoidance of the secondary infection.

1. Bed rest
2. ● Mouth washes — Tetracycline (*see* page 42)
    ● Chlorhexidine gluconate mouth wash 0.2%; 10 ml 2–3 times daily.
    ● Miconazole oral gel, 25 mg per ml, applied to the affected mucosa after food.
3. Systemic antibiotics. Penicillin V elixir or Erythromycin elixir 250 mg 6 hourly.

2. Secondary herpes

The most common site for recurrent herpes is on the lips although it may occur within the mouth or anywhere on the face. The lesion begins as a series of vesicles which soon rupture, and is followed by crusting extra-orally and coalescing ulcers intra-orally. Herpes simplex infection recurrs in otherwise healthy people when they are subjected to other disease (cold sore), emotional upset or exposure to sunlight. It is a frequent complication in patients who are immunosuppressed.

Management. Acyclovir 5% in aqueous cream base; apply four hourly for five days. Idoxuridine 5% in dimethyl sulphoxide, apply four hourly for five days.

For treatment of children see also p. 96.

Erythema multiforme

This is a systemic disease mainly affecting young adults and may be recurrent. It may follow some ten days after a respiratory tract infection, but has been associated with many viral and bacterial infections, particularly herpes simplex. Drug hypersensitivity and hypersensitivity to certain preservatives in food have been implicated. It commences with malaise and a low pyrexia, with bullae appearing rapidly, usually over a period of 24–36 hours. It may involve the mouth only, but similar lesions may occur on other mucous membranes, the conjunctiva or genitalia, and over almost any part of the body surface. The severe form of the disease is known as Stevens-Johnson syndrome.

The oral lesions characteristically involve the lips and gingivae but the whole oral cavity may be involved. There is local lymphadenopathy and extreme pain and discomfort, so severe as to make even the taking of fluid almost impossible. The bullae soon rupture leaving enormous erosions. The lips become crusted and bleed readily; this is said to be characteristic of the condition.

Management.
1. Bed rest
2. Mouth washes as for ulcerations
3. Systemic steroids — prednisolone 60 mg per day in divided doses reducing to nil within ten days, can abort an early recurrent attack or cure an established disease within three to four days. Systemic steroids should only be given under the direction of a physician.

Herpes zoster (Shingles)

This condition, caused by a reinfection with varicella (chickenpox) may reveal itself first by pain (*see* Chapter 1). It can affect any dorsal root ganglion and the trigeminal ganglion. If it affects the second or third division of the trigeminal nerve, vesicles and/or bullae will develop on the skin and mucous membranes within the area supplied by that division. It is rare that two divisions may be involved simultaneously. Lesions present as red circumscribed areas about 2–10 mm in diameter developing 36–48 hours after the onset of pain. Initially they may be well circumscribed but, particularly on mucous membranes, may become confluent and soon rupture releasing millions of virus particles. The ruptured vesicles become encrusted on the skin but in the mouth they form ragged painful ulcers with healing taking a week to ten days. The lesions are accompanied by pyrexia, general malaise and sometimes profound depression.

Management.
1. *Bed rest*. This is essential to reduce complications and allow rapid recovery.
2. *Parenteral fluid replacement*. If the pain from the oral lesions is severe. The patient would require referral to hospital for treatment.
3. *Systemic antibiotics*. These may be required to reduce secondary infection. For example, Ampicillin 250 mg four times per day for five days, or Metronidazole 200 mg three times per day for five days.
4. *Oral topical antibiotics* may be helpful where the mucous membranes are involved. Miconazole gel and tetracycline mouth washes are the most beneficial (*see* p. 42).

Usually the younger patient recovers rapidly and completely. With advancing years, patients tend to have a protracted course. Additionally, the elderly are prone to suffer post-herpetic neuralgia for which no effective treatment has been devised.

Pemphigus

This takes many forms but the acute condition is the most common of the variants. The condition overall is uncommon and may involve either sex in late middle to old age. It is an autoimmune disease where the cement substance of the suprabasal layers of the epithelium is affected, causing intraepithelial bullae. The result is a sloughing of the skin and mucous membranes and, due to fluid loss and electrolyte disturbance, can become rapidly fatal. On the skin it can be characterized by the rapid appearance of vesicles and bullae which may start only a few millimetres in size but may spread rapidly and coalesce over large areas of the skin. Often it appears first in the mouth, where its development is less dramatic. The correct diagnosis is important as it may herald the development of the skin manifestations. The bullae arise generally in the unattached gingivae, and the mucosa of the floor of the mouth and cheek. Bullae develop rapidly and soon form ragged ulcers with a tendency to bleed when touched. A characteristic feature of pemphigus is that the epithelium at the edge of the ulcer may be picked up and stripped from the adjacent oral mucosa. This is known as the Nikolsky sign. A dental napkin run over apparently normal mucosa, will create a similar ulcer with the epithelium being stripped away. The lesions are exquisitely painful.

Management. If pemphigus is suspected, particularly where a Nikolsky sign has been elicited, immediate referral by telephone to a department of oral medicine/oral surgery or dermatology should be made. It is imperative that the diagnosis must be made definitively and rapidly so that treatment may start so as to prevent skin lesions developing. Before the advent of corticosteroids and anti-metabolites, the condition was fatal.

Pemphigoid

This is a benign chronic bullous condition, affecting the mucous membranes and the skin. The lesions never would create an emergency except with its possible confusion with pemphigus. It is an auto-immune condition with the bullae made up of entire epithelium, the split being in the sub-basal layers, creating subepithelial lesions. Thus, the blisters are generally robust and difficult to strip away from the underlying tissue. It more commonly affects females with the oral lesions involving the gingivae and the junction of the hard and soft palate. It is painful and unpleasant, although the inflammation is far less marked than pemphigus. The lesions seldom bleed. The bullae eventually rupture and may leave raw eroded bleeding surfaces. Healing is slow.

Management. It is important to differentiate pemphigoid from pemphigus and thus if the clinician is unsure of the diagnosis a referral by telephone to a hospital department of oral medicine/oral surgery or dermatology should be made so that an early definitive diagnosis may be made . Treatment with topical steroid preparations may help to remove the discomfort but the condition is characterized by remissions and exacerbations generally out of medical control.

Angina haemorrhagica bullosa recurrens

This is a rare condition, only recently recognized, where patients present with painful blood-filled blisters, which appear within minutes and may reach up to 1 cm in diameter. Occasionally the blisters rupture early and cause bleeding from the mouth although this is seldom severe. Predominately, it affects females of any age. A crop of blisters may form, commonly on the soft palate and fauces, and collapse within hours leaving ragged ulcers. They heal within a few days, but may recur regularly in various parts of the mouth, probably as a result of trauma. The cause is unknown.

Management. There is no specific management for this condition but referral to hospital is important so that a bleeding diathesis can be excluded.

Vitamin B$_{12}$ deficiency

Severe vitamin B$_{12}$ deficiency which has been allowed to remain unrecognized may be accompanied by bullous lesions of the oral mucosa which have distinct similarities with the lesions of pemphigus. However, the usual signs of B$_{12}$ deficiency will be apparent, with extreme macrocytic anaemia, debility and confusion.

Bear in mind: the possibility of Vitamin B$_{12}$ deficiency, when called to see an elderly confused female in an Old Persons' Home who has large, apparently painful ulcers and bullae on the oral mucous membranes.

III PURPURA AND TELANGIECTASIA

Purpura is a blue/grey discolouration of the mucous membranes (and also skin) due to a spontaneous extravasation of the blood within the tissues. Usually the extravasation is confined to multiple small spots 1–2 mm in diameter over any part of the mouth. Frequently it is symptomless. Generally the causes of this rare condition are a deficiency in the blood clotting mechanism, particularly a decrease in the number of platelets, or deficient platelet activity. It can be due to capillary fragility.

Thrombocytopenic purpura

A reduction in the number of circulating platelets may be primary (idiopathic) or secondary to other disease (bone marrow replacement, eg. leukaemia, severe toxic states, autoimmune disease). The favoured site for the oral lesions are over the soft and hard palate. Purpura frequently represents a bleeding tendency, and the commonest oral manifestation is profuse gingival haemorrhage, particularly where there is pre-existing gingival inflammation.

Management. If a cause for the purpura has not been diagnosed previously, an urgent referral to hospital is required. In those with established purpura, attention must be paid to achieving good gingival health. Gingival manipulation and extraction of teeth should only be carried out with the agreement of the physician in overall charge of the case.

Hereditary haemorrhagic telangiectasia

This uncommon condition can resemble purpura. It is a rare hereditary condition where telangiectases develop late in life, particularly in the oral mucous membranes. Raised red swellings 2–3 mm in diameter appear particularly on the palate but also on the other oral mucous membranes, and can bleed readily when traumatized. The patient may be unaware of the lesions until they bleed. Examination of the mouth will reveal a small number of telangiectases, with one of them bleeding uncontrollably.

Management. Usually direct pressure fails to control the bleeding, and thus more active measures are required. Local anaesthetic solution containing adrenaline should be infiltrated into the area and the bleeding point cauterized. This can be done with a hot instrument or diathermy. Referral to a hospital department of oral surgery and oral medicine is advised for further investigation and treatment of the remaining telangiectases.

IV   WHITE PATCHES

White patches seldom develop rapidly and therefore they are unlikely to be considered an emergency by a clinician. However the patient may notice them for the first time and become anxious about them. The only white oral lesion to have an acute onset associated with inflammation, is that due to *Candida albicans.*

Acute candidiasis

This can affect all age groups, but the acute form occurs generally in the young. When it does occur in adults, it is usually in patients debilitated by systemic disease.

Raised white soft plaques appear over a part or all the oral mucosa, with favoured sites being the buccal and lingual tissues. The plaques may spread to the lips, particularly to the angles of the mouth. Each plaque measures up to 5 mm in diameter and may be rubbed off leaving a bleeding base. The patient will complain of generalized soreness of the mouth. An infant or child may have a pyrexia and be anorexic. Secondary infection in the lesions may lead to cervical lymphadenopathy.

Management
1.   Topical anti-fungal agents are usually successful. Miconazole oral gel 25 mg per ml applied to the mouth, preferably after careful oral hygiene, three times a day and on retiring.
2.   Amphotericin as a suspension (100 mg/ml) or preferably as lozenges, 10 mg, dissolved in the mouth slowly three times a day and on retiring.
3.   Nystatin as a suspension or preferably tablets, containing 500,000 units dissolved slowly in the mouth three times a day and on retiring.

A five day course of any of the above is usually sufficient.

The following conditions should be borne in mind

1.   Oral candidiasis may be a marker for systemic disease and/or local mucosal abnormality:

General disease
- Diabetes
- Leukaemia
- Wasting diseases
- Dehydration, particularly as seen in old age.

Local disease
- Dysplastic lesions — leukoplakia, erythroplakia.
- Carcinoma
- Chemical burn (rare) caused by aspirin or similar substance which has been held adjacent to a tooth which is painful.

2. Candidal lesions on the floor of the mouth, side of the tongue, at or behind the angles of the mouth, should be examined thoroughly and biopsied to exclude underlying malignant disease.

3. Candidiasis or thrush frequently is diagnosed in error for other white lesions seen in the mouth and listed below. While the organism may be present in the mouth and be identified in many white lesions, it is seldom the primary cause of white lesions in adults. *Always* consider the following before making a diagnosis of oral candidiasis —

   (a) *Lichen planus* — a relatively common condition seen predominantly in middle-aged females, affecting primarily the buccal tissues from the posterior molars forwards. It may affect the gingivae or tongue, but seldom in isolation. Characteristically it has a lace-like pattern with fine radiating white lines extending out from the periphery of the lesion. Central areas may break down to form ulcers, particularly in the cheeks and sometimes on the tongue.

   (b) *Hyperkeratosis* — raised white areas, usually much larger than that caused by thrush, on an uninflamed base in keratinized mucosa subjected to recurrent trauma. This is never seen in the floor of the mouth.

   (c) *Leukoplakia* — this is a white patch of varying size and shape arising from dyskeratotic epithelium, for which no other diagnosis may be ascribed. It may occur anywhere in the mouth and is generally considered to be pre-malignant. The most dangerous areas are the lateral border of the tongue and the floor of the mouth. Any white patch seen in these sites should be referred to a department of oral surgery or oral medicine.

   (d) *Hairy leukoplakia* — the white patches appear to be hairy forming strands coming out from the lesion. While rare at present, it is seen exclusively in acquired immune deficiency syndrome (AIDS) and is likely to be on the increase. Specialist consultation must be arranged.

4. *Erythema migrans* (Geographic tongue). This relatively common condition results in migrating red patches on the tongue where the filiform papillae become deficient. Frequently, adjacent to the

red areas the papillae lengthen and a white halo results. It is a condition noted for its exacerbations and remissions. The depapillated areas become tender, particularly to spicy and astringent foods. The discomfort and appearance make the patient fearful that the condition is serious and an urgent consultation is requested. The patient should be reassured as to the benign nature of the condition.

V   THE LIPS

Lesions and inflammation of the lips are usually associated with disease within the mouth or systemic disease, and thus careful intra-oral inspection is always mandatory. Nonetheless there are problems which seem to be restricted entirely to the lips.

Angular cheilitis

Inflammation at the corners of the mouth may be a local entity but also aggravated by systemic disease. The infecting organisms causing the inflammation will be mixed but *candida albicans* and *staphylococcus aureus* prominate. Examination of the mouth may show old, ill-fitting dentures causing overclosure. There may be evidence of chronic candidiasis.
A careful history should be taken to exclude systemic disease such as diabetes, leukaemia and the blood dyscrasias.

Management. The areas should be dried and an anti-fungal preparation applied (Miconazole gel 25 mg per ml, Amphotericin ointment or Nystatin ointment). An anti-staphylococcal preparation may be equally effecive (Fusidic acid ointment). Ointments are better than creams as they tend to be water repellent.

Cracked lips

This is a familiar winter problem frequently associated with habitual licking of the lips when out in cold weather. With children the inflammation may spread beyond the vermillion border. In the adult a persistent cracking of the lips may occur with scarring, so that the lesion may remain in the same place; it bleeds on stretching and can be very painful if secondarily infected.

Management. For the child, a simple barrier cream, or even petroleum jelly may suffice. For the adult with a persistent crack in the lip, Betamethasone ointment to reduce inflammation is helpful in the acute stage, but should not be used more than three times a day over a period of a week.

Bear in mind: a persistently cracked lip in the adult may represent malignant change, particularly if it occurs in the lower lip.

In a younger patient with thickening and cracking of the lips, consider the possibility of Crohn's disease.

Swollen lips

Sudden diffuse swelling of the lips may occur as a result of allergy or hypersensitivity to certain antibiotics, particularly Penicillin. It seldom occurs alone and usually is associated with other signs such as a rash or general oedema of the face. Antihistamines may be helpful but the underlying cause of the swelling must be sought. If extreme or persistent, referral to an allergy clinic is recommended.

An unusual condition, the Melkersson-Rosenthal syndrome, is associated with swelling of the lips and partial facial nerve palsy. This is extremely rare.

Bear in mind: the feeling of swelling of the lips is a common symptom in elderly people. If no swelling is seen, it is likely to be part of the oral dysaesthesia complex. In this condition, the patient complains of a combination of a burning tongue, dry mouth, a bad taste and sometimes stringy saliva — and swollen and burning lips. Reassurance is all that is required.

VI   RED MOUTH

This is more a sign than a symptom and may be noted at oral examination. If there are symptoms of soreness other possible causes listed above should be excluded. When symptoms are few and the redness is restricted to the denture-bearing area, the causal organism is likely to be *Candida albicans*. In part the infection is related to bad oral and denture hygiene, which allows the ingress of *candida* into the mucosa and prosthesis. Improved oral hygiene must be encouraged, and anti-fungal preparations such as Miconazole gel, Amphotericin or nystatin cream may be applied to the fitting surface of the denture, after meals and on retiring, with a denture worn until the next meal is taken. It is necessary usually to construct new dentures, once a cure is established. Subsequently, it is important to advise patients not to wear their dentures at night, and to place them in water to which a mild disinfectant such as sodium hypochlorite has been added.

Bear in mind:

1. Patients who are suffering from iron deficiency are more susceptible to mucosal infection by *Candida albicans*.
2. Candida ingress may herald systemic disease such as diabetes.
3. In the floor of the mouth, candida ingress may be the marker for dyskeratotic or malignant mucosal change.
4. Isolated red/blue swellings up to 1 cm in size may represent Kaposi's sarcoma, a marker for acquired immune deficiency disease.

VII   TEETHING

Teething is an uncomfortable experience for every child. It is a pericoronitis around erupting teeth and is self-limiting, seldom needing treatment. Where a pyrexia develops it may be necessary to give systemic antibiotics such as penicillin V elixir. Topical medicaments, such as Bonjela rubbed into the sore areas, may be helpful.

6: Medical Emergencies

All dental practices must be properly equipped to deal with any emergency which might be anticipated to occur during treatment. Sudden loss of consciousness is one such emergency. A list of equipment and drugs which should be available at all times in the dental surgery is seen in Table 6.1. There must be ready access to all

Table 6.1 Emergency equipment for the dental surgery

I EMERGENCY OXYGEN

There *must* be a source of oxygen in every practice. If the premises are not on a single floor, the emergency oxygen apparatus must be portable or there must be one available on each floor. You cannot be expected to carry an anaesthetic machine up stairs particularly at a time of crisis.

The apparatus should be a 170 litres, size C, oxygen cylinder. A reduction valve, rebreathing bag (Amubag) and face mask must be fitted. A key for opening the valve on the cylinder must be attached to the apparatus. There should be an oro-pharyngeal or Brook airway.

The cylinder(s) must be checked regularly by a representative of the British Oxygen Company and they must be replaced when nearly empty.

II EMERGENCY MEDICATION

An emergency box complete with the necessary medication can be obtained from many sources. It is most important that the practitioner is aware of the various procedures rather than have to rely on the directions in the box.

The shelf life of each of the medications has to be checked and the medications replaced as necessary.
The box should contain:
- Vials of adrenaline tartrate injection BP (1 : 1000 adrenaline)
- 2 bottles of 100 mg hydrocortisone sodium succinate injection.
- 2 × 10 mg ampules Chlorpheniramine maleate (Piriton)
- 2 cc ampoules of Sterile water for injection.
- 50 ml glucose injection strong BP 50% w/v
- Glucagon hydrochloride 1 mg
- 4 vials diazepam BP 10 mg in 2 ml for i.v. injection
- 2 × 200 cc sterile disposable syringes
- 2 × 2 cc sterile disposable syringes
- Butterfly canula 21 gauge needle

this equipment, and the dental nurse, and all those working in the practice, must know where it is kept. All the chair-side assistants, and preferably the receptionist(s) too, should be familiar with contents of the emergency box, and be trained for the emergency situation. The equipment should be checked monthly, and outdated drugs replaced.

I THE UNCONSCIOUS PATIENT

As soon as the patient is found to be unconscious:

1. Lay the patient flat, preferably on the floor. If consciousness is lost while in a dental chair, adjust it so that the patient's head is lower than the feet initially, until a diagnosis is established.
2. Establish an airway with a custom-made tube, such as a Brook airway. If this is not immediately available, extend the neck and protrude the mandible by pushing forwards against the vertical ramus. Check that there is a wide-bore tip in the aspirator.
    If the patient becomes unconscious and these facilities are not available, for instance if the patient is in the waiting room or hallway, turn the patient on the side and extend the neck, and call for assistance.
3. Attempt to detect a pulse at the carotid.
4. Look for signs of spontaneous breathing by observing chest movements.
5. *Note the time accurately.*
6. If there is no sign of spontaneous breathing and a pulse cannot be detected after 90 seconds from the estimated time of loss of consciousness, commence cardiac massage. This is best carried out with the patient on the floor (*see* Table 6.2). Call for as much local assistance as possible, and instruct one of the helpers to summon an ambulance immediately.
7. If there is a pulse and spontaneous breathing, *stop and think.* Establish a diagnosis.

Faint

This is the most common cause of loss of consciousness in the dental surgery. It is the result of a reduction in blood supply to the brain, and cerebral hypoxia. The most frequent cause is anxiety and, during

Table 6.2   Cardiorespiratory arrest

1. Establish the diagnosis — check the carotid pulse; note respirations.
2. Summon as much help as possible.
3. If the patient is not on a dental chair or firm couch, lay him on the floor. Elevate the legs.
4. Thump the chest — a clench fist hit hard over the lower part of the sternum.
5. *Note the time accurately.*
6. Summon as much assistance as possible.
7. Insert a Brook airway and fit a self-inflating (e.g. Ambu) bag.
8. Commence external cardiac massage — place both hands, one on top of the other, over the lower end of the sternum (*not over the heart*). With the arms straight, put your weight down over the chest as if to squeeze the chest wall against the vertebral column. It is a smooth, not jerky, movement. Do this approximately once per second.
9. Ventilate at approximately 15/minute using the bag, or mouth-to-mouth.
10. Check for the return of a normal pulse at frequent intervals.
11. Check the diameter of the pupils at frequent intervals. If there is a progressive dilatation, the patient's condition has a poor prognosis.

In hospital:

12. Set up an intravenous line.
13. Infuse 100 ml of 8.4% sodium bicarbonate immediately, and follow this with normal saline.
14. Insert a cuffed endotracheal tube.
15. Set up an ECG.

Maintain the circulation and respiration until skilled assistance arrives.

---

dental treatment, the most common time for it to occur is during or shortly after an intra-oral injection, or after a procedure is completed. It is more likely to occur in those who have a low blood sugar and those who give a history of fainting. Such faints may be prevented by ensuring that the patient has eaten before arriving at the surgery, and by arranging for all procedures to be carried out with the patient in the horizontal position.

Some medical conditions make the likelihood of fainting greater:

1. Cardiac arrhythmias — uncontrolled heart block (detected by a pulse less than 50 per minute in the unfit), those prone to transient ventricular asystole (Stokes-Adams attacks), and those treated within 3 months of a myocardial infarction.
2. The hyertensive patient taking ganglion-blocking drugs (unusual now). Some patients with severe disease of the nervous system, such as disseminated sclerosis, will be prone to fainting if the autonomic nervous system is involved. There is no danger in

treating these patients provided that such treatment is carried out with the patient in the horizontal position.
3.   In the anaemic patient.

Management. Wait for the return of consciousness and, as appropriate, consider continuing treatment after discussion with the patient.

If there is a possibility that the loss of consciousness could be associated with underlying disease, discontinue treatment and seek medical advice.

Occasionally, a faint may be followed by a convulsion. This tends to occur if the faint has been prolonged and is caused by cerebral hypoxia. It does not however, mean that the patient is epileptic, but precautions should be taken to protect the patient from damage during the seizure.

Epileptic fit

There are two common forms of epilepsy, grand mal and petit mal. Petit mal will result in unconsciousness but without convulsions and no apparent loss of control. The patient, if upright, may not even lose balance, appearing merely to have a vacant expression for a few moments. Grand mal usually results in convulsions with loss of co-ordination. Both forms of epilepsy are generally self-limiting and all that is required is to wait until consciousness returns.

Management. Recovery from a petit mal attack is rapid, and no special precautions need to be taken. If dental treatment has been started, it may continue.

Management of a grand mal attack is as for the unconscious patient, set out above. It is important to remove all loose objects from the mouth, particularly complete dentures, and to protect the tongue from damage. A Brook airway is ideal. The clonic stage seldom lasts more than a few minutes and is followed by drowsiness which may last minutes to hours, during which the patient may have slurred speech, complain of a headache and feel generally unwell. Each patient is usually well-versed in what he or she is able to do in the post-convulsion phase. If dental treatment has been started, it should be curtailed.

Rarely, in the unstable epileptic, seizures may be prolonged or follow one another in rapid succession. Should this happen, with clonic phases lasting more than 10 minutes, medical advice should be sought or an ambulance summoned. Epileptic attacks lasting more than 30 minutes (status epilepticus) are dangerous as the hypoxia and hyperthemia may lead to brain damage. Should the requested help not be forthcoming at this stage, benzodiazepines stored in many practices for intravenous sedation, may be used. Diazepam or midazolam 10 mg given slowly i.v. may well abort an attack. While larger doses are sometimes required, seek medical advice before giving more than this amount.

Avoidance of an attack. Well-controlled epileptics can be treated just like any other patient with no special precautions. Generally, it is wise to ensure that the patient is treated within 90 minutes of eating and, if the patient is very nervous, is given additional sedation before arriving at the surgery.

Febrile convulsions in children

Infants and children up to the age of 5, suffering an acute infection causing rapid temperature rise, may suffer convulsions. This could happen during 'teething' — pericoronitis associated with erupting deciduous teeth, or an acute periapical abscess.

Management. Take and record the temperature at the axilla. Remove as many clothes from the child as possible to assist rapid cooling. Usually it is necessary to explain to the mother or father that the fit is due to excessive temperature, for it is their natural reaction to keep their child warm when it is sick. Sometimes it is necessary to cool the child further with a fan if cooling is not rapid enough. Once the child has stopped fitting, replace only enough clothes to keep the child warm, and refer to the patient's medical practitioner, by telephone.

Prescribe antibiotics to contain the causative infection — penicillin V or erythromycin elixir 125 mg four times per day.

Diabetic coma

Diabetics patients may become unconscious from hyperglycaemia, or hypoglycaemia. Hyperglycaemia is slowly progressive over hours or days, while hypoglycaemia may be abrupt and dangerous, requiring decisive and immediate action.

1. Hypoglycaemia

The diabetic patient may be receiving insulin injections or pills (sulphonyl ureas) for control of their condition. Some may be controlled by diet alone, and will not be at risk from hypoglycaemia. Those requiring insulin injections are less stable than those taking hypoglycaemic agents, and are more likely to become hypoglycaemic. An experienced patient will recognize the symptoms:

- (a) He will feel hungry
- (b) He will be irritable
- (c) He will be aware that he is at risk — for instance, he may well have missed or be late for a meal.

There will be other signs of which he may not be aware:

- (d) He will be excitable, irrational and may be disoriented. He may be aggressive and give the appearance of being drunk. Before calling the police, consult your notes and consider that he may be a hypoglycaemic diabetic.
- (e) If unconsciousness follows, examine for a tachycardia, dilated pupils and moist skin.

Management

1. If the patient is conscious, persuade him to take a glucose drink. Orange juice with added sugar would be a good alternative.
2. If the patient progresses rapidly to unconsciousness, inject glucagon 1 mg i.m. This will raise the blood sugar to within the normal range within a few minutes, by mobilizing the liver glycogen. An ampule of glucagon should be available in every dental surgery.
3. As soon as the glucagon has been given, seek medical help.

Bear in mind: if in doubt, administer the glucagon. This will do no harm.

2. Hyperglycaemia

The approach of coma, through pre-coma, is slow, and may take a day or so. If a severe infection is present, it may approach in a matter of hours and thus may be recognized in the dental surgery. The signs will be as follows:

- (a) The patient will have been becoming increasingly drowsy.
- (b) There will be signs of water depletion — a dry slack skin, hypotension with dizziness on standing, and tachycardia. There will be a history of polyuria.

(c) There will be signs of acidosis — deep sighing respirations with perhaps a foetor of ketosis.

Management

- Hyperglycaemic pre-coma or actual coma does not represent a great emergency, unlike that from hypoglycaemia. If there is doubt as to which the diabetic is suffering, give oral glucose as above, for it will do no harm to the hyperglycaemic diabetic, but can save the hypoglycaemic patient from real damage.
- If infection has been the precipitating factor, ensure that this is being treated adequately.
- Refer the patient to the medical practitioner immediately by telephone.

There is no hazard in providing dental treatment for a diabetic who is well-controlled. The normal dose of insulin or hypoglycaemic agent should be given and normal food taken. There is some advantage in treating the patient early in the day because diabetic control is generally at its best at this time. Infections destabilize the blood sugar, and must be treated immediately and rigorously should they occur.

Stroke

Loss of consciousness due to a stoke (cerebrovascular accident) is likely to be exceedingly rare in the dental surgery. It may be caused by haemorrhage, thrombosis or embolism. Although the incidence of stroke is greatest in the elderly, the patient does not necessarily have to be old. The rupture of a vascular malformation in the brain (berry aneurysm) can occur from late puberty onwards. It is precipitated by transient high blood pressure. This might occur in the very stressed and nervous patient. The signs of stroke vary according to the site of the lesion in the brain. There will be:

(a) Profound unconsciousness
(b) The eyelash reflex will be absent. (Running a finger across the eyelashes will not produce a blink reflex)
(c) Eye movements — generally nil. There may be inappropriate rolling movements
(d) Pupils — variable according to site of lesion. Unilateral dilatation suggests raised intracranial pressure and urgent transfer to hospital
(e) Respirations — generally normal
(f) Limbs flaccid in the early stages.

Management

1. Lay the patient flat
2. Aspirate to clear secretions from the mouth
3. Insert a Brook airway
4. Administer oxygen
5. Call for medical assistance and/or ambulance.

Occasionally the effect of a stroke may be transient, and the patient may not even become unconscious. This is known as *transient ischaemic attack* caused by microemboli or a sudden decrease in blood flow to the brain, both occurring in atherosclerotic vessels. The patient may become confused and have temporary loss of function of a limb or loss of clear speech. The signs will vary according to the site of the ischaemia in the brain.

Such attacks may herald a full cerebrovascular accident and the patient must attend his general practitioner urgently or be referred directly to hospital.

II CHEST PAIN

Differential diagnosis

1. Myocardial ischaemia or infarction
2. Hiatus hernia, with reflux oesophagitis
3. Tracheitis
4. Pulmonary disease — pleurisy, pulmonary infarction
5. Dissecting aneurysm.

Myocardial ischaemia and infarction

Angina presents as a pain centred upon the chest and is identical to that for myocardial infarction (see below) except that it is self-limiting, lasting for minutes only. It is precipitated by stress, with the typical patient being an overweight, cigarette-smoking male who has hurried on a cold day to keep the dental appointment for which he is late. Anticipation of painful dental treatment may be the final precipitating factor.

The presentation of myocardial infarction is variable. The younger patient presents with more dramatic and severe symptoms than the older patient, whose symptoms are less determinate.

Clinical features

(a) Sudden severe crushing pain in the chest. Radiation down the arm is frequent, with the left arm the more commonly involved. Occasionally, radiation may be to the neck and mandible. Rarely, the pain may present primarily in the mandible or arm with little central chest discomfort.

(b) The pulse may be slow with irregularities in rhythm (ectopics). Where there is an arrhythmia present, treatment is required urgently.

(c) There may be hypotension. Remember that a previously hypertensive patient may appear to be normotensive when examined after a heart attack.

(d) The patient may feel faint or giddy, or complain of palpitations. In the elderly, this may be the only presentation.

Without ECG and tests for cardiac enzyme changes it is difficult in some cases to make a diagnosis. In the 'at risk' group (overweight, smoking, family history of cardiac disease) and where the patient has had a history of angina, assume that there is a myocardial infarct.

Management. If the pain is thought to be angina, give the patient trinitrotoluene (TNT) to be dissolved under the tongue. If the pain does not resolve quickly:

1. Lie the patient flat. A dental chair is ideal, but if the floor is the most convenient place, let it be the floor. Support the head and make the patient as comfortable as possible. Do not choose a sofa or deep armchair, for if cardiac arrest occurs, resuscitation is difficult or impossible.
2. Call assistance in case there is need for emergency resuscitation.
3. Instruct a member of staff to summon an ambulance, giving the ambulance control your provisional diagnosis. Some districts have ambulances equipped for cardiac emergencies.
4. Do *not* give the patient any beverages.
5. A few patients may go rapidly into congestive cardiac failure, and this can lead to pulmonary oedema. If there are signs of respiratory embarrassment, lift the patient into a semi sitting position.
6. Be prepared to give external cardiac massage and artificial respiration (*see* Table 6.2, page 57).

Hiatus hernia

The chest pain is felt centrally and at the base of the sternum. It may spread over the lower chest and never refers down the arm. If the reflux is more extensive, it may result in 'heart burn' or pain bubbling up to the throat. Gastric reflux into the mouth may be experienced, and then the diagnosis becomes obvious. It is unlikely that there will be other signs of bradycardia, extrasystoles etc., suggesting a cardiac origin. The patient may well recognize the pain.

Management. Sit the patient up and as far as possible reduce all external pressure upon the abdomen by releasing the waist band, clothes etc. Oral antacids are helpful.

Tracheitis

This is a central chest pain which should present little difficulty in diagnosis. The patient will have signs of an upper respiratory tract infection with a 'dry' cough. The pain may be described as 'raw', behind the sternum, and worse on coughing. A more lateral chest pain exacerbated by coughing and deep breathing, might represent pleurisy. The anxiety with which some people present at the prospect of dental treatment or when they have experienced some pain at the hands of the dentist, can cause hyperventilation (*see* page 68) and an accentuation of the pain.

Other causes of chest pain

1. Pulmonary embolism
2. Pneumothorax
3. Dissecting aneurysm
4. Pericarditis.

Management. Lay the patient face down, give oxygen if available, and call medical assistance or an ambulance. Nurse the patient in a sitting position if there are signs of heart failure with dyspnoea and production of a frothy, blood-stained sputum.

III SHOCK

Anaphylaxis and anaphylactic shock

Anaphylaxis may occur within minutes of a dose of drug to which the patient is sensitive, and may progress to shock. *Always* ask a patient, before administering any drug, whether or not there is a known allergy to it. Anaphylaxis may occur with no previous history of allergy and the onset may not be immediate. It may develop after the patient is no longer on the premises.

Signs

1. Generalized itching of sudden onset
2. Sudden urticaria
3. Flushing
4. Acute anxiety.

These may be taken as the warning signs and there may be no further progression. However, if not arrested, the progression will be:

5. Wheezing
6. A feeling of constriction in the chest with laboured breathing.
7. Abdominal pain, nausea and vomiting
8. Circulatory collapse
9. Death.

Management

1. Lay the patient horizontal
2. Inject adrenaline 1:1000 solution slowly *intramuscularly* to combat shock, at the rate of approximately 1 ml/min. If this were to be injected subcutaneously rapidly in the shocked patient, it will not be absorbed sufficiently fast due to peripheral circulatory failure. There is no risk of causing ventricular fibrillation *provided that* the injection is deeply intramuscular and aspiration before injection indicates that a vessel has not been punctured inadvertently. This should be injected at 15 minute intervals until improvement occurs.
3. Inject hydrocortisone succinate 200 mg i.v. to suppress further allergic response.
4. Inject chlorpheniramine maleate (Piriton) 10–20 mg i.m. to reduce further histamine release.
5. Administer oxygen.
6. Call for medical assistance and/or an ambulance.

Bear in mind: if the patient, having left the premises, telephones and describes symptoms and signs suggesting anaphylaxis, advise that the medication be discontinued and that, should the condition worsen, an ambulance should be summoned immediately.

Adrenocortical insufficiency

For all practical purposes, an Addisonian crisis is only likely in patients already taking steroids on a long-term basis. The pituitary-adrenal axis is suppressed or may be completely atrophic, and cannot respond to additional demand.

Clinical findings — consider the following:

(a) The patient is on steroids, has been for at least a year and is likely to be carrying a steroid card.

(b) The patient may lose consciousness, but this will be slowly progressive and will not be as dramatic as a faint. There will be hypotension and the patient may be nauseated or even vomiting.

(c) There is likely to be evidence of increased metabolic demand. Infection, particularly dental abscess, is the most common cause, but consider myocardial infarction or stroke. It is most unlikely that routine dental or oral surgical procedures under local anesthesia could be responsible, unless infection is present sufficient to induce a bacteraemia.

(d) There may be signs of dehydration — a creased, lax skin of the forearm, which fails to flatten after gentle pinching.

Management

1. Place the patient in a horizontal position. Be prepared to tip the head lower than the feet and pelvis if the blood pressure is not restored rapidly.

2. Aspirate the mouth to clear the airway if the patient should vomit. The patient is likely to be sufficiently conscious to maintain the airway in normal circumstances.

3. Give hydrocortisone succinate 200 mg. i.v.

4. Call for medical assistance and/or an ambulance.

5. Set up a drip of normal saline at a rate of 1 litre in two hours, if available.

The presentation may not be as dramatic as described above. The patient may just feel unwell, nauseated, and a little dizzy on standing from a sitting position. If the predisposing factors described above are present, double the oral dose for that day.

IV RESPIRATORY

Hyperventilation and tetany

It is not an infrequent occurrence in the dental surgery, that a nervous patient becomes distraught. As anxiety escalates overbreathing occurs, and the patient becomes aware of physical changes which make the panic worse and increase the hyperventilation. This creates hypocalcaemia as carbon dioxide is removed and the blood becomes relatively alkaline.

Clinical findings

(a) A frightened, restless patient, more commonly a young female
(b) Obvious hyperventilation
(c) Tingling of the fingers which spreads also to the feet and circumoral parasthaesia.
(d) Carpopedal spasm, where the fingers are pulled together in flexion. In extreme cases, the wrists become flexed and the body hunched. The patient experiences cramp-like feelings and interprets the experience as a spreading paralysis, and the panic worsens.
(e) Occasionally the patient may lose consciousness.

Management

1. Attempt to persuade the patient to rebreathe from a paper or polythene bag. This is not as easy as it sounds, for the patient, already thinking that the end is nigh, finds that the dentist is attempting to smother him or her! Firm, calm persuasion usually wins the day, followed by massive reassurance.
2. If this fails or is impossible, diazepam or midazolam 7–10 mg i.m. will control the situation in a few minutes. For more rapid action, this may be given intravenously, but patient anxiety makes venipuncture difficult.
3. Once the patient is calm and is able to understand, discuss the events which led to the crisis, and explain their significance.

Bear in mind: hyperventilation can be the sign of salicylate overdose. Do not confuse an acute asthma attack with hyperventilation; intravenous or intramuscular sedation may increase the hypoxia.

Asthma attack

The most likely cause of breathlessness in an asthmatic is an acute asthma attack. Anxiety, particularly in a child, may precipitate an acute asthmatic episode, as can infection or allergy. It is wise to avoid treating an emotional asthmatic who is recovering from a chest infection, or in that individual's bad time of the year for allergic asthma.

Clinical findings

(a) Severe dyspnoea, with the patient becoming too breathless to speak.

(b) Evidence of airway obstruction — laboured breathing, pronounced wheeze, and use of the accessory muscles of respiration. Occasionally, so little air may be moved that wheezing is not apparant.

(c) Tachycardia in excess of 120/min.

(d) Cyanosis.

Management

1. Double the dose of the patient's usual inhaler. This may not succeed and therefore progress immediately to the following:

2. Inject hydrocortisone succinate 200 mg i.v. immediately, and add oral prednisolone, with an immediate dose of 20 mg.

3. Administer oxygen.

4. Call medical help and an ambulance.

Bear in mind: never give adrenaline because the patient may have been prescribed a β_2 adrenoceptor stimulant (for example, salbutamol as an inhalant).

7: Management of HIV and Hepatitis B (HBV) Patients

Every patient must be considered as a potential carrier of HBV, because most carriers are undiagnosed. If the patient presents with acute hepatitis A or B infection, (i.e. he is jaundiced) treatment should be carried out in a hospital. Patients who belong to the 'high-risk' groups should be identified from the medical history.

Patients who are chronic carriers of hepatitis B or are shown to have HIV infection (positive antibody test but not debilitated) may be treated by the General Dental Practitioner (GDP) if the following precautions are taken in general practice:

1. *All dental personnel in clinical contact with patients should be vaccinated with vaccine (H-B-Vax) against HBV.*
2. Take a sound and thorough medical history of each patient and update it regularly.
3. Use disposable material and equipment where possible. Cover all working surfaces with 'Cling-film' *not* paper because when paper becomes wet it is no longer impermeable.
4. Ensure that all non-disposable instruments are thoroughly cleaned and then sterilized by autoclave.
5. The wearing of gloves, masks, gowns and spectacles for the operator and assistant is mandatory.
6. Ensure that the aspiration equipment exhausts external to the confines of the building.
7. Make sure that all impressions are thoroughly rinsed under running water and placed in 2% glutaraldehyde (Cidex) for a minimum of ten minutes before sending them to the technician (this will *not* sterilize the impression but will disinfect it). Advise the technician to wear gloves while handling the impressions and casts poured from them.
8. Place all waste in rigid sealed containers or sealed plastic bags. There must be a separate 'sharps' container.

If patients offer the information that they are an HIV or an HBV carrier, it is important to conform to the above procedures and in addition:

9. Arrange the appointment at the end of the day.
10. Protect the equipment controls and handles of the operating light with cling film.
11. *Do not use* ultrasonic instrumentation or the airotor so as to avoid contamination from the aerosol.
12. Take exceptional care to avoid needle stick injuries.
13. Make all impressions in silicone material and soak in 2% glutaraldehyde for three hours.
14. Disinfect all working surfaces with hypochlorite solution.
15. Flush the aspirator with 2% glutaraldehyde and leave overnight.
16. Launder the gowns at 90°C for 10 minutes if disposable gowns are not available.
17. Incineration of all disposable items must be arranged.

The booklet *Guide to Blood Borne Viruses and the Control of Cross Infection in Dentistry* published by the British Dental Association is highly recommended as a guide to this problem.

8: The Dentist's Responsibility in Cases of Suspected Child Abuse

In 1983, in England and Wales, 700 *identified* deaths of children under 16 were due to child abuse, and six in every thousand children under the age of 16 were found to have suffered abuse at the hands of an adult or adults.

The dentist has no more duty to report the incident or to protect the child than any other member of the community. The general statutory responsibility for care and protection lies with the Local Authority who can invoke care proceedings in the Magistrates Court.

The Police and the NSPCC have powers to bring care proceedings but not the duty to do so.

Any person, but usually the police, may apply to a Magistrate for a 'place of safety order' which, if granted, runs for a maximum period of 28 days. The police may also detain a child in a place of safety without prior application to a court and can obtain powers of entry in the course of action to protect a child.

The responsibility of the dentist

The General Dental Practitioner (GDP) is in a position to identify families under stress which might put a child at risk from abuse, or to notice if a child is being abused. The practitioner has responsibilities to both the parent and the child as dental adviser, but also to the child as a protector.

Any information must be shared with the statutory services responsible for the child's protection, namely the police, the NSPCC and the social services. The practitioner's knowledge of the family will also contribute to any subsequent assessment of the child in court proceedings.

It is most important to remember that most abused children return to the family home even if removed for an initial period.

Signs and recognition of general abuse

It is unlikely that the parents will present a child to the GDP immediately following injury for fear of being found out; the GDP being regarded as part of the overall medical team.

It should also be remembered that physical abuse is only one aspect of child abuse. Others such as physical neglect, emotional abuse, and in particular sexual abuse, are more difficult to recognize. An abused child may be of any age or from any social background.

The common sites for the everyday *accidental* injury are the forehead, the occiput, bony spinal protuberances, the elbow, iliac crest, knees and shins, but the sites for *non-accidental* injuries are the eyes, ears, cheeks, mouth, neck, shoulder, upper arms, inner arms, and the front and back of the thighs. Consider the following with suspicion:

1. Black eyes are suspicious if both eyes are black (most accidents cause only one), the eyelids are swollen and tender, there is no bruise on the forehead or nose, and where there is a suspicion of a skull fracture.
2. Bruising in or around the mouth especially in small children. This can be accompanied by a tearing of the labial frenum of the sub-lingual frenulum as a result of a feeding bottle or other implement being forced into the mouth with excessive force. If this is continued over a long period of time, the lower front teeth can be damaged or retroclined.
3. Symmetrical bruising particularly of the ears, 'outline bruising' for example in the shape of a hand or linear bruising on the hands or arms should be noted. In normal circumstances children will fall forwards and acquire one or two bruises to bony prominences. Usually there will be signs of damage to the palms of the hands if they have tried to break their fall.
4. Human bite marks are oval or crescent shaped. If the distance across the oval or crescent shaped impression is more than three centimetres, they must have been caused by an adult or older child with permanent teeth. If possible take photographs of the bite marks with a millimetre scale rule adjacent to the lesion in the picture.
5. Burns and scalds are difficult to differentiate as being accidental and non-accidental burns and scalds, but as a general rule burns or scalds with well defined outline of a uniform depth and which cover a large area should be regarded with suspicion. Always look for evidence of previous injury.
6. All children have scars but notice should be taken of an exceptionally large number, differing age scars, unusually shaped

scars from lacerations or burns which did not receive medical attention.
7. Physical neglect should be suspected if the child is of short stature and underweight for his/her age. The skin is cold and exhibits pink/purplish mottling. Limbs may be swollen and have slow healing pitted sores. The hair may be dry and sparse and there may be signs of alopecia. The child may have a 'pot-belly'. Often he/she may stay frozen in one position for an unnaturally long period of time, apathetic and unstimulated by their surroundings.

The GDP could become involved in child abuse incidents which take place on his premises and which demand urgent attention. It is more likely that the practitioner recognizes or suspects that abuse has occurred and non-urgent management has to be considered.

ACTION IN THE SURGERY

1. Non-urgent action

It may not be possible to write up the notes while the child or the parent are in the surgery. The notes must be completed as soon as possible and in great detail. Be careful to note the clinical findings, conversations and events pertinent to the case. This information must be reported in writing to the appropriate authority, e.g. police, social services, over the next few days. Your notes will have to be made available to the court if legal proceedings follow.

If possible take photographs without arousing the suspicion of the parent or parents. Ask the child how the injuries were acquired and then ask the parents. Note any obvious differences in the explanations. Note the site and nature of the injuries and the date on which they were observed.

If child abuse is suspected, contact the Social Services Office which is appropriate for the address of the family. This can be found in the local telephone directory. Pass on the information taken above; this should be followed up in writing within the next few days. Ask the Social Services Office to tell you if the name of the child or any other child of the family is on the 'At Risk Register'.

2. Urgent

If you are witnessing actual abuse taking place on your premises, telephone the local Police Station and the Youth Community Bureau.

The Police have powers to remove the child from the surgery in the event of an emergency.

Follow up these events in writing over the next few days.

ACTION ELSEWHERE

If there is cause for concern, the Social Services will hold a case conference. They may ask the GDP to attend, but if this is not possible any observations can be made in writing.

If court proceedings are taken, the letters of the Dental Practitioner may be produced and he/she may be called as a witness. The parents of the child are not usually present at a case conference but usually they will be present in the court.

FOLLOW-UP ACTION IN THE SURGERY

Note any abuse or suspected abuse on the patient's record card and link these records with those of any siblings. Also make a note on the record card if the child's name is on the local 'At Risk Register' and also link this information with the records of the siblings.

Make notes on the records of the outcome of any court proceedings.

9: Restorative Emergencies

The most frequently occurring emergencies are discussed in different sections of the book. These are:

- Irreversible pulpitis (*see* Chapter 1, page 4)
- A fractured or lost restoration (*see* Chapter 1, page 6)
- A fixed bridge which has become uncemented on one abutment tooth
- Pin penetration of pulp
- Lateral perforation of a root
- Vertical root fracture (*see* Chapter 3, page 34)

I PROBLEMS FOLLOWING THE PLACEMENT OF A RESTORATION

Once a restoration has been placed the following conditions may occur:

- Thermal sensitivity
- Gingival discomfort
- Discomfort to biting on the restoration
- Problems associated with inadequate approximal contacts
- Galvanic reactions
- Cervical sensitivity

Thermal sensitivity

This may be the consequence of the method of preparation itself. Preventive measures should have included an adequate amount of coolant in the correct place on the bur, adequate thickness of dentine over the pulp or proper pulp protection, care not to dessicate the exposed dentine and the placement of adequate lining material. Occasionally the placement of pins may produce thermal changes due to conduction along the pins themselves or the crazing of the dentine between the pins.

The acid etch procedures associated with composite materials may produce severe post operative discomfort if the dentine has not been protected completely during the etching process or if the composite resin restoration has not been completely cured.

Management. Remove the offending restoration and place a sedative dressing such as zinc oxide/eugenol. If pins have been used as part of the restoration these must also be removed. Carefully explore the floor of the preparation for evidence of a pulpal exposure or a crack. If a pulpal exposure is found to be present, root canal therapy should be initiated. If the pin holes are too close together and microcracks in the dentine are suspected, line the floor of the preparation with calcium hydroxide and seal it in with a glass ionomer cement.

Gingival discomfort

This might be related to the placement of a matrix band or retraction cord, the presence of an overhang on a restoration or the retention of a foreign body, e.g. a piece of retraction cord, a piece of a wooden wedge or some impression material in the gingival crevice.

Management. Traumatic injuries to the gingival tissues respond well to being left alone. Hot salt mouthwashes and analgesics such as paracetamol may help.

Attempt to find a foreign body, but this is often difficult because the tissues bleed profusely on probing. Curettage of the gingival sulcus will remove any offending remnants.

Where an overhang is present it is sometimes possible to remove it with an ultrasonic scaler otherwise the restoration must be removed and the preparation dressed with a provisional material, such as a well contoured zinc oxide/eugenol dressing. This allows the gingival tissue to return to a state of health before replacement of a definitive restoration.

Discomfort on biting

This may be due to either a high restoration, or a crack in the tooth which has been made worse by the restorative procedure.

Management. A high spot in intercuspal position may be identified easily on an amalgam or cast gold restoration by noting the presence of a burnished area. This must be adjusted making sure that the holding cusp contact (that contact maintaining the occlusal vertical relation in the intercuspal position) is retained. High spots in the intercuspal position on porcelain restorations may be more difficult to identify and often articulating paper does not mark the surface. Where these high spots appear on holding cusps of porcelain restorations, try to retain the integrity of the glaze by making the adjustment in the opposing fossa. If the adjustment has to be made on the porcelain, careful finishing and polishing is mandatory. Problems arise if the masking porcelain (kernmasse) of a ceramo-metal crown is exposed because this cannot be glazed and will produce severe wear of the opposing tooth or restoration, and remaking the crown on a modified preparation should be considered.

It is important to assess occlusal contacts in all excursions, especially when the anterior teeth are involved although the inter-cuspal contacts may be satisfactory, these interferences only become evident when the patient moves into an excursion. The displacement of the tooth may be felt easily by palpation. Place a finger on the labial surface of the tooth and ask the patient to move the mandible into the excursion which would be most likely to displace the tooth. Adjustment must be confined to the palatal aspect of the upper anterior teeth and the temptation to adjust the lowers should be avoided.

When a cracked tooth is suspected, remove the restoration. If a piece of the tooth comes away with the restoration fit a protective provisional crown. Glass ionomer cements are useful in this situation. If the crack cannot be located the tooth should be dressed with calcium hydroxide sealed in with a suitable temporary filling material (*see* Chapter 1, page 7).

Problems associated with inadequate approximal contact

(a) *Open contact*: this is often associated with the plastic restorative materials such as amalgam, particularly if a spherical alloy has been badly handled. Posterior composites are notorious in this respect because they do not have the viscosity to resist the tension of the matrix.

Management. Remove the restoration and replace, ensuring a sound contact area. It is possible sometimes to key a piece of restorative material into the existing restoration as a temporary measure (a stop-gap procedure!).

(b) *Tight contact*: this happens usually following the cementation of a crown or bridge rather than the placement of a plastic material. The patient complains of a feeling of having something between the teeth, or that the text are being pushed along the dental arch.

Management. If possible, remove the restoration and adjust the contact area. If this is not possible or impractical the contact can be opened using a wedge and the contact area adjusted with polishing strips. This is a difficult and unsatisfactory procedure.

Galvanic restorations

The usual complaint is of sensitivity similar to that which occurs when biting accidentally on a piece of 'silver paper'. It occurs when restorations of dissimilar metals contact in the presence of saliva. It may occur between gold and amalgam and even between new amalgam and old amalgam. The latter may occur when an old amalgam restoration is 'patched'.

Management. Often all that is required is reassurance that the reaction will gradually diminish with time. In severe cases an application of ammoniacal silver nitrate, neutralized with eugenol over the offending restoration greatly decreases the discomfort. This procedure *must* be carried out under rubber dam.

Cervical sensitivity

This problem may present before any restorative procedures are carried out or as the result of placing a cervical restoration, particularly a Class V acid etched composite restoration.

Management. If a recent restoration is the cause, this must be removed and a sedative dressing (such as zinc oxide/eugenol) placed. The management of cervical sensitivity is dealt with in Chapter 1, page 9.

II PROBLEMS OF EXISTING CROWNS AND FIXED BRIDGEWORK

Apart from endodontic considerations (*see* Chapter 10, page 87) the more common problems associated with crown and bridgework are:

- Fractured porcelain from an anterior bonded crown or bridge
- Uncemented crowns
- Crowns which have dislodged due to fracture of the preparation
- Uncemented post crowns
- Fractured posts
- Uncemented bridge retainer
- Broken solder joint of a fixed bridge
- Gingival irritation under a pontic

Most of the emergency procedures for these conditions require removal of the crown or bridge and the fabrication of provisional crowns or bridges. Suggested methods are as follows:

Acrylic provisional crowns

1. Select a provisional anterior crown form of the correct size (celluloid, or better still polycarbonate).
2. *Apply liberal amounts of petroleum jelly to the preparation.*
3. Mix some reline material (e.g. Sevriton) and over-fill the crown form by a small amount.
4. Wait until the reline material has just reached the initial set.
5. Cover the surface of the unset reline material with petroleum jelly and seat the relined crown form on the previously lubricated preparation.
6. Remove and replace the provisional crown until the reline material begins to set and heat up.
7. Place the provisional crown in hot water until the reline material is set. Trim off the excess with an acrylic bur. If a celluloid crown form has been used, peel it away from the acrylic.
8. Re-try the provisional crown on the preparation and adjust for length and any interferences in all mandibular excursions.
9. Polish the margins and any adjusted surface with a soft white rubber wheel.
10. Cement the provisional restoration with a provisional cement such as Temp-Bond.

Provisional bridges

1. Make an alginate or silicone impression of the damaged bridge after reconstituting any damaged area with wax or acrylic (Duralay).
2. Remove the damaged bridge and *lubricate the preparations well with petroleum jelly.*
3. Mix a provisional bridge material (e.g. Pro-Tem) and load it into a disposable syringe.
4. Inject the material into relevant areas of the impression ensuring that the nozzle of syringe is buried in the material as it is expressed. This avoids air entrapment.
5. Seat the impression in the mouth until the material is set. It is useful to place a little of the material on the handle of the impression tray as a guide to the degree of setting.
6. Remove the tray and the provisional bridge.
7. Trim off any excess and take care to ensure that the fit surface of any pontic conforms to a modified ridge lap contour and that all embrasure spaces are open. (It may be of assistance to mark the margins of the retainers with pencil before commencing the trimming.)
8. Check and adjust for interferences in all mandibular excursions.
9. Polish the margins, any area which has been adjusted and the fit surfaces of any pontic.
10. Cement the provisional bridge with a provisional cement such as Temp Bond.

Fabrication of a provisional bridge where the original is not available

Sometimes a provisional bridge has to be made when an original is not available to copy. In such circumstances a provisional bridge has to be sculptured from a block of acrylic.

1. Refine the margins of the preparations and *lubricate the preparations and the occlusal surfaces of the teeth opposing the provisional bridge with petroleum jelly.*
2. Mix sufficient provisional bridge material (e.g. Sevriton).
3. Apply petroleum jelly to the finger tips and mould the acrylic into an oblong shape, long enough to incorporate both abutment teeth and the space between them.

4. Place the unset resin over and between the preparations moulding it to the prepared teeth.
5. Ask the patient to close into the intercuspal position and then to open. Remould the material to the preparations, because the contact of the teeth tends to pull the soft acrylic away from the preparations.
6. When the acrylic commences the final set, remove and place it in hot water.
7. Trim off the excess material from the margins and shape the material freehand to replace the retainers and the pontics.
8. Once it has completely hardened, mark the margins of the preparations and the approximate widths of the various retainers and pontics with pencil.
9. Try in the provisional bridge and adjust interferences in all mandibular excursions. Finally polish every surface.
10. Cement the provisional bridge with a provisional cement (e.g. Temp Bond).

Fractured porcelain

If a porcelain jacket crown fractures remove the remnants and fabricate an acrylic provisional crown.

If porcelain fractures from an anterior ceramo-metal crown use either:

(a) one of the proprietary 'porcelain repair kits' (such as Kerr Command Ultrafine Repair Bonding System) following the manufacturer's instructions asiduously.

or

(b) remove the crown completely and make an acrylic provisional crown.

Unless the appearance is compromised and there are no sharp edges, there is usually no real problem when porcelain fractures away from posterior fixed bridgework. The patient must be reassured that it is the metal subframework which can be seen and that the natural tooth is protected.

When porcelain fractures from anterior ceramo-metal bridgework the result will be a compromise of the appearance. Attempts at making a repair using a 'porcelain repair kit' may be tried, but often the only satisfactory method is to remove the bridge and fabricate an acrylic provisional.

Be very careful to ensure that during the removal of a ceramo-metal restoration all pieces of loose porcelain are accounted for and immediately removed from the mouth with the aspirator.

Uncemented crowns

When there is a failure of the luting cement of a crown the restoration is not necessarily displaced from the preparation. This is particularly common when a single retainer of a bridge becomes uncemented. Complaints of sensitivity on biting and temperature changes may be apparent if the tooth has not been root filled. In most instances the patient will complain of an unpleasant taste and a tendency of the gingival tissue to bleed.

The crown appears mobile and pressure on the occlusal surface will produce bubbles of saliva from the margin.

Management. Remove the crown and clean both the fit surface of the crown and the preparation. Confirm that there is no fracture of the tooth or root and no exposure of the pulp.

Check the seating of the crown, the proximal contact areas and the occlusal contacts in all excursions. Examine for obvious occlusal interferences. Make the necessary adjustments, repolish the surface and recement the crown.

Crowns which have dislodged as a result of fracture of the preparation

The method of replacement will greatly depend on the condition of the remainder of the preparation. Two periapical views taken from different angles will be necessary to assess which treatment options might be considered.

Management. If sufficient dentine covers the pulp and the margins of the crown still fit, two small pins may be placed into the root face and the crown reseated using a glass ionomer cement. Care must be taken to fill the crown completely and to ensure that the root face is covered completely with the cementing medium.

If insufficient coronal dentine remains, carry out elective endodontic therapy and replace the existing crown using a provisional post. The provisional post may be made of a piece of stainless steel wire (paper clip!) or a preformed post may be used (Parapost system).

A provisional post crown using stainless steel wire and self cure acrylic may be made as follows:

1. Remove part of the new root filling and prepare the canal to accept a provisional post.
2. Lubricate the canal with glycerine and blow the excess away using air.
3. Place the provisional post in the canal. Try in the crown over the post to ensure that it seats fully. Bend the coronal portion of the wire bent into a loop to give retention for the acrylic. Adjust the length of the post until the crown seats fully. If no crown is available use a polycarbonate provisional crown
4. Fill the crown with self cure acrylic (Sevriton), and place some in the entrance of the root canal.
5. Make notches in the stainless steel wire and introduce it, or the preformed post into the canal. Fill the crown with self cure acrylic and seat it over the post.
6. Remove the excess acrylic from the gingival margin. Partially remove and replace the crown until the acrylic is set. Remove the crown from the tooth and place it in hot water to accelerate the set of the material.
7. Trim away the excess acrylic. Re-try the crown on the tooth. Check the occlusion in all mandibular excursions and adjust any interferences.
8. Polish the margins and any areas which required adjustment. Seat the provisional post crown with a provisional cement.

If it is possible to complete the elective endodontics at the one visit, a preformed post (Parapost) can be cemented into the canal and the core built up immediately.

If the root should have fractured below the crest of the alveolar bone and orthodontics is not thought to be appropriate, extract the root.

Uncemented post crowns

One of the most common causes for a post crown to become uncemented is a vertical fracture of the root. This can be confirmed by inserting a wide, blunt instrument (flat plastic, ball ended burnisher) into the post canal and GENTLY try to elicit the separation of the fragments. If the root is intact remove any retained cement from the post crown and from the canal. Recement the post crown.

Fractured posts

Fractured posts have to be carefully drilled out or attempts at removal may be made using a Masseran Kit (*see* Chapter 10, page 90) if available. Ultrasonic devices (Cavitron) may also be of help. If removal is successful fabricate a provisional post crown. If these procedures fail extraction may be the only course of treatment.

Where it proves impossible to replace the crown immediately; in many instances the anterior appearance is compromised. Consider the following:

1. Add a tooth to an existing partial prosthesis.
2. Fabricate an immediate partial prosthesis if laboratory facilities are available.
3. Attach a denture tooth (or even the crown of the patient's natural tooth if available) to the neighbouring teeth with an acid etch procedure. The patient must be warned that this will be a weak attachment.
4. Place pins in the proximal surfaces of the neighbouring teeth and attaching a denture tooth with self cure acrylic or an acid etch procedure. This is only recommended if the definitive restoration involves the crowning of these teeth.

Uncemented bridge retainers

It is very important to recognize that a bridge retainer has become uncemented because caries may rapidly destroy the underlying preparation. The patient may complain of sensitivity to biting and temperature changes. The condition may be recognized by applying pressure to the occlusal surface of the suspect retainer and observing the cervical margin. If bubbles of saliva are expressed from this area the retainer is uncemented.

Management. Attempts must be made to remove the bridge. The patient should be warned that the bridge and the abutment teeth may be irreversibly damaged. Frequently the bridge has to be cut off, repaired and remade. If the bridge is damaged beyond repair a provisional bridge has to be made using one of the procedures described above.

Broken solder joints

Broken solder joints tend to occur in long span, fixed-fixed bridges or in ceramometal bridgework where there has been insufficient interproximal height for adequate thickness of metal to be placed. If these were designed correctly, the metal framework would be brought to the occlusal surface of the bridge and 'compromise the appearance'.

Management. In the short-term see if it is possible for the bridge to survive in its present state, or if the broken joint can be repaired with self cure acrylic. If it is considered that either part of the broken bridge could compromise the appearance or the integrity of the abutment teeth, the bridge must be removed. A provisional bridge may be constructed using one of the techniques described above.

Gingival irritation proliferation under a pontic

The fault lies in the design of the pontic which may prevent proper cleaning or encourage a piece of food debris to become trapped beneath the pontic. The gingival tissue is very swollen, erythematous and bleeds easily.

Management. Attempt to remove any foreign material with dental floss. Severe bleeding usually occurs. Prescribe Corsodyl mouthwash. If the condition recurs repeatedly, the bridge must be removed.

10: Endodontic Emergencies

VERY IMPORTANT

Inhalation or swallowing of an endodontic instrument may be avoided if proper precautions are taken. In the unfortunate event of this happening the patient *must* be told and *must* be sent for a chest and/or abdominal radiograph. The Medical Protection Organization *must* be informed immediately.

The best form of protection is prevention

Use rubber dam in all endodontic procedures

I EMERGENCIES BEFORE ENDODONTIC TREATMENT IS COMMENCED

The most common endodontic emergencies which occur before treatment are:

- Pulpal pain
    - (a)   reversible pulpitis
    - (b)   irreversible pulpitis
- Acute periapical abscess (*see* Chapter 2, p. 16)
- Pulpal exposure as a result of a fracture (*see* Chapter 3, p. 33)
- Cracked tooth syndrome (*see* Chapter 1, p. 7)

Bear in mind: other conditions can present similar signs and symptoms, e.g. TM joint dysfunction, periodic migrainous neuralgia, maxillary sinusitis, cervical spondylitis, etc.

Pulpitis

1. Reversible pulpitis (*see* Chapter 1, p. 6 and 7)

The patient complains of discomfort on taking hot, cold and sweet food. The pain lasts several seconds and the offending tooth is difficult to locate. Electric pulp tests give an early response, the tooth is not necessarily tender to percussion, radiographs show no changes in the supporting tissues and the colour of the tooth is normal.

Management. Remove the cause, for example a deep or faulty restoration. Seal a calcium hydroxide dressing in the tooth with zinc oxide/eugenol dressing.

2. Irreversible pulpitis (*see* Chapter 1, p. 6)

The patient complains of pain which is spontaneous, initiated by heat and may last for minutes or for hours. At first the offending tooth is difficult to locate but becomes very tender to percussion.

Management. Remove the pulp. Place the rubber dam, prepare an adequate access cavity and remove the pulp tissue and debris using files and copious amounts of hypochlorite solution in a disposable syringe. Dry the canal with paper points. Seal the access cavity. It is recommended by some to seal a hydrocortisone/antibiotic paste (Ledermix) into the pulp chamber.

Acute periapical abscess (*see* Chapter 1, p. 16)

The affected tooth becomes mobile and very painful to touch and to heat although cold may relieve the discomfort. The pain decreases as a swelling appears. The swelling is diffuse at first but becomes fluctuant and points. The patient will develop a pyrexia at some stage.

Management. Open the pulp chamber with a round bur in an air rotor using light pressure. Usually local analgesia is not necessary but if it is required do not infiltrate into the infected area, but use regional analgesia. If no pus or discharge drains from the root canal pass a size 15–20 file through the apex. Endodontists suggest this is the only situation when the apex should be penetrated deliberately.

Place the rubber dam. Irrigate with copious amounts of sodium hypochlorite solution and dry the canal with paper points. Seal the access cavity and relieve the tooth from the occlusion. If the discharge cannot be controlled, leave the access cavity open for 24 hours. Reassure the patient and prescribe analgesics and antibiotics. (Amoxycillin 3 g sachet followed by amoxycillin capsules 500 mg three times a day for four days commencing eight hours after the sachet has been given.)

If there is a fluctuant swelling which is pointing intra-orally, particularly associated with the mandibular teeth where drainage through the root canal may not be adequate, incise at the most fluctuant point.

If the abscess is *fluctuant* extra-orally but *not pointing* refer to the nearest department of Oral Surgery, by phone if there is a pyrexia.

Often, complete debridement is not possible especially in molar teeth where there may be three or four canals. In such instances a pulpotomy should be performed. Remove the pulp tissue from the pulp chamber with a large, sharp excavator. Place a pledget of cotton wool impregnated with metacresyl acetate (Cresatin) without pressure into the pulp chamber. Seal the abscess cavity with a provisional restoration.

Cracked tooth syndrome (*see* Chapter 9, p. 77)

The symptoms of the patient depend on the degree of involvement of the pulp tissue. The tooth is tender to bite on and pulpitis, progressing to periodontal pain occurs. There may be mobility of the two fragments of the tooth.

Fractured teeth (*see* Chapter 3, p. 33)

II EMERGENCIES DURING THE TREATMENT

Inadequate analgesia

This may arise when there is an acutely inflamed pulp. Regional and/or infiltration analgesia are ineffective. The standard techniques may be supplemented with intraligamental injections and intrapulpal infiltration.

Where these techniques are still ineffective, the exposed pulp tissue may be dressed with a corticosteroid paste (Ledermix) sealed in with a temporary dressing material. This is a temporary measure and the patient must be told that the pulp will have to be extirpated at a later appointment. The patient may be reassured that the problem with analgesia probably will not recur.

Fractured endodontic instrument

Inform the patient that the instrument has fractured in the tooth. Explain that it may still be possible to complete the root filling satisfactorily. The Masserann Kit may be used if available, in an attempt to remove the fragment. This consists basically of a hollow bur which cuts the dentine around the fractured instrument so that it may be more easily engaged and removed.

The fracture of files and reamers may be prevented by discarding old or damaged instruments, progressing correctly through the sizes during canal preparation, not rotating them more than one-half a turn and never forcing the instrument into the canal.

Perforation of a root

This is a particular danger when gaining access to the root canal of a tooth which has been restored with a full crown. Often the alignment of the crown and the root are dissimilar. If perforation does occur, it is advisable to thoroughly clean the canal if possible and fill completely with calcium hydroxide paste (calcium hydroxide BP mixed with local anaesthetic solution). Ensure that the access cavity is properly sealed. An acid etch composite resin material is useful for this.

Incomplete canal preparation

Discomfort may occur if all pulpal remnants are not removed from the canal(s). All canals must be cleaned to the apex.

If signs and symptoms persist, this may be due to the presence of an *extra canal* which has not been located. Upper and lower first molars may have four canals, lower canines and incisors two canals; often the lower first premolar may have two canals but the lower second premolar rarely has two canals. Locate the accessory canal and clean.

III   EMERGENCIES FOLLOWING ENDODONTIC TREATMENT

High restoration

Locate the interference on the temporary restoration and adjust.

The following complications will require that two periapical radiographs, at differing angles be taken to assist in making a correct diagnosis.

Infected pulp tissue or debris left in the canal

Remove the root filling and clean the canal to remove any remaining infected material. Consider the possibility that there may be an additional canal. If it proves impossible to remove the root filling, consider apicectomy or extraction.

Root fracture

Usually this is a vertical fracture and tends to occur following the placement of posts in the roots of small teeth. Extraction is the only possible treatment.

Underfilling

Where possible attempt removal of the root filling and clean out the residual root canal at the apex. If the root filling is poorly condensed it is relatively easy to remove. Clean the canal properly and reseal.

Overfilling

It is very difficult to remove root fillings which extend beyond the apex unless the material is a silver cone or a poorly condensed gutta percha point. A reasonable assessment of the material used may be made from the radiographic appearance of the root filling. If it proves impossible to remove, prescribe analgesics (aspirin, paracetamol or BUPROFEN). Sometimes apicectomy or even extraction has to be performed particularly when the root filling material is a paste which has extruded through the apical foramina.

IV EMERGENCY ENDODONTIC TREATMENT IN THE PRIMARY DENTITION

While every attempt must be made to retain the primary teeth until they are exfoliated, sometimes extraction is necessary. Removal of anterior primary teeth has few orthodontic implications but the posterior primary teeth serve an important function to maintain space for the permanent dentition. When extraction is unavoidable always consider the possibility of doing balanced extractions.

All the procedures available for the treatment of pulpal involvement in the primary dentition involve the use of calcium hydroxide. If there is caries deep into the dentine and an exposure is suspected, seal calcium hydroxide over the caries free dentine with a temporary cement (indirect pulp capping).

If there is evidence of a small pulpal exposure on a non-infected pulp, cover with calcium hydroxide (direct pulp capping), line the cavity and place a permanent restoration.

Sometimes it is possible to remove the coronal pulp and leave the radicular pulp (vital pulpotomy). Cover the exposed radicular pulp tissue with calcium hydroxide and seal into place. This technique is carried out in an attempt to keep the radicular pulp vital so that the formation of the apex of the root is completed.

Bear in mind:

- This type of treatment is very useful for treating first permanent molars in children.
- If there is uncontrollable haemorrhage from the radicular pulp, complete extirpation must follow because it must be assumed that the infected process has progressed to involve the radicular pulp tissue.
- Where it is not possible to obtain complete analgesia, expose the coronal pulp and apply paraformaldehyde on a pledget of cotton wool to the pulp tissue. *Do not apply pressure*. Place a soft layer of provisional dressing over the medicament to seal the access cavity.
- The patient and the parents must be warned that there might be discomfort for a few days for which analgesics may be necessary. The patient must be seen for review in one or two weeks.

11:   Periodontal Emergencies

The most common periodontal emergencies are:

- Abscess formation
  - (a)   Periapical abscess
  - (b)   Periodontal abscess
  - (c)   Gingival abscess
  - (d)   Combined perio/endo lesion
- Acute marginal gingivitis
- Acute necrotising ulcerative gingivitis
- Acute herpetic gingivo-stomatitis
- Self inflicted gingival and mucosal injuries
- Gingival swellings of systematic disorders
- Periodontal surgery: post-operative problems

Abscess formation

Often it is very difficult to differentiate the cause of an abscess. It may be pulpal or periodontal. The management of a periapical abscess is given on page 16 and that of a periodontal abscess on page 17.

The diagnosis is made from the information gleaned from:

- History of pain as described by the patient. A deep dull ache, not affected by temperature changes is suggestive of a periodontal abscess. The tooth can be uncomfortable to bite on with either pulpal or periodontal pathology. The dental history may help if it reveals that a large restoration is present, or if endodontics or periodontal therapy has been recently carried out.
- Clinical examination can be inconclusive because a discharging sinus may be present with either of these conditions in the later stages. Generally, if the periodontal condition is good and the problem involves an isolated tooth then the cause is likely to be of pulpal origin.
- Vitality tests can be inconclusive especially if the tooth has been heavily restored.

- Probing of the gingival crevice may reveal a pocket but a periapical abscess can discharge through the gingival sulcus.
- Radiographs are not conclusive although careful examination of the integrity of the lamina dura can be of assistance.
- Problems occur if the lesion is related to the furcation area of multi-rooted teeth because this is often the site of a combined perio/endo lesion.
- One of the most useful tests if an abscess is discharging through the gingival crevice or through a sinus, is gently to insert a gutta percha endodontic point into the affected crevice or sinus and take a radiograph of it in position. If the lesion is a periapical abscess the point will travel to the apex of the offending root.
- As a general rule if a combined periodontal/endodontic lesion is suspected, commence root canal therapy, because this would be the first procedure to be completed whether the lesion be an endodontic or a combined lesion.
- State of general health. A periodontal pocket which has been inactive can become acute during the course of some systemic disorder which reduces the resistance of the patient's tissues.

Gingival abscess is dealt with on page 18.

Acute marginal gingivitis

This condition may not be an emergency for the practitioner but it may well be so for the patient. The clinical sign which concerns patients is the spontaneous bleeding from the tissues which they believe might be due to an aggressive systemic complaint.

Management. Confirm the diagnosis clinically and reassure the patient by explaining the cause and preventive measures. Commence the removal of plaque and calculus. Instruct the patient on hygiene control and stress the importance of follow-up visits. Antibiotics usually are not required.
Bear in mind: spontaneous bleeding from the gingival tissues can arise as a result of atrophy in 'desquamative gingivitis', erosive lichen planus, mucous membrane pemphigoid and acute myeloid leukaemia.

Acute necrotising ulcerative gingivitis

History: the patient complains of mild to severe pain in the gingival tissues usually accompanied by difficulty with eating, has 'bad breath' and a nasty metallic taste in the mouth. There may be a history of spontaneous gingival bleeding, pyrexia and cervical lymphadenopathy. In many cases the patient is a smoker and often under stress.

Clinical examination: there is a characteristic foul odour to the breath. Ulceration is restricted to the gingival margin with necrosis of the gingival papillae which have a punched-out appearance. There may be a grey pseudomembrane over the tissues.

Management. Debride and irrigate as well as possible remembering that this is an uncomfortable procedure for the patient. Prescribe Metronidazole 200 mg three times a day for five days. Hydrogen peroxide mouthwash 20 vols, diluted 1 : 4 may be helpful. Ensure patients understand the importance of returning for appointments with their general dental practitioner.

Acute herpetic gingivostomatitis

Usually seen in infants and the symptoms occur abruptly. The complaints are of pain, increased salivation and halitosis. The infant is very irritable. There may be cervical lymphadenopathy and marked pyrexia.

Clinical examination reveals a grey-yellow membrane surrounded by bright red mucosa. All mucosal surfaces are involved.

Management. Prescribe Acyclovir (Zovirax) 100 mg five times a day at four hourly intervals for five days if the patient is under two years of age. If over two years of age prescribe 200 mg five times a day at four hourly intervals for five days.

Self inflicted gingival and mucosal injuries

(a) Toothbrush trauma: Over-vigorous toothbrushing in an area where there is thin gingival tissue over a bony prominence is probably the most common cause. A toothbrush with splayed filaments may also be a factor.

Enthusiastic use of dental floss can cut the gingival papilla and give rise to a gingival abscess.

Management. Explain to the patient what has happened. Allow the lesion to heal for one week and suggest that during this period the patient cleans the plaque from the teeth rather than 'scrubbing the gums'. (Immediately send a letter making peace with the patient's periodontist.) Suggest that the toothbrush is replaced.

Trauma may be inflicted also by overzealous flossing and the incorrect use of interdental stimulators. Careful demonstration of the correct procedure is required.

(b) Chemical injuries: Patients may apply topical agents, such as oil of cloves, aspirin and other medications to the gingival tissue and mucosa in the belief that this may reduce the discomfort. This may produce localized epithelial sloughing.

Bear in mind: stomatitis artefacta, *see* page 40.

Management. Identify the offending agent, counsel and reassure the patient; also identify and treat the reason for the original need to use the agent.

Gingival swellings of systemic disorders

Gingival swellings can occur locally and generally. Isolated local swellings include a periodontal abscess, pyogenic granuloma and a pregnancy epulis.

General swelling of the gingival tissues can be a result of drug induced hyperplasia (from phenytoin or cyclosporin). Rarely, it may be as a result of acute myeloid leukaemia.

Periodontal surgery: post-operative problems

(a) Postoperative infection

Symptoms throbbing pain, swelling and even cellulitis begin about 48 hours after the surgery, and the clinical signs must be differentiated from postoperative swelling. Examine for cervical lymphadenopathy and take the patient's temperature.

Bear in mind: the possibility of pulpal problems requiring endodontic therapy.

Management. Establish drainage of the infection which may entail the removal of the periodontal pack and even the sutures. Advise the patient to use hot salt water mouthwashes hourly. Prescribe antibiotics only where there are systemic symptoms. Where the infection is associated with a loosened periodontal pack, renew it.

(b) Postoperative bleeding

This may occur as a result of postoperative infection, inadequate suturing, a loosened periodontal pack, or a combination of the three. Spontaneous bleeding may sometimes occur; if this happens within the first 24 hours post-operatively it is unlikely to be due to infection.

Management. In all cases, stop the bleeding by pressure over the pack. The use of local anaesthetic solution with a vasoconstrictor is sometimes required. If necessary suture under local anaesthetic. If associated with infection or to the pack becoming loose, remove the pack, irrigate and debride as required and renew the periodontal pack. If there are signs of systemic spread prescribe metronidazole 200 mg three times a day for five days or penicillin V 250 mg four times a day for five days.
Bear in mind: patients who are on anticoagulant therapy.

(c) Dentine hypersensitivity

This may persist following periodontal surgery or as the result of localized recession, and is most acute where pulpal hyperaemia has been associated with existing restorations.

Management. No really effective means of control has yet been discovered (except endodontics!) however the severity may be reduced with fluoride mouthwashes, (En-de-Kay 2% sodium fluoride), topical steroid application (Adcortyl-A paste), and other desensitizing agents (Duraphat).

12: Prosthodontic Emergencies

Prosthodontic emergencies may be related to:

- new complete dentures
- fractured complete dentures
- immediate replacement dentures
- fractures in partial dentures
- immediate additions to partial dentures.

It is often impossible to correct a problem with a prosthetic appliance using a 'stop gap' procedure. A further appointment will usually be required when the facilities of a dental laboratory are available.

Immediate repairs may sometimes be carried out if plaster and self curing acrylic are available. The cause of a fracture must be determined and corrective measures employed to prevent further emergencies. For example, a complete upper denture might fracture in the midline as a direct result of the base rocking on the midline of the hard palate. Although the fracture may be repaired, unless the fit of the base is adjusted the fracture will recur.

NEW COMPLETE DENTURES

Problems with new complete dentures can present as:

(a) generalized inflammation
(b) localized bruising and ulceration related to the denture bearing mucosa
(c) localized bruising and ulceration related to the periphery
(d) palatal ulceration
(e) cheek biting

Generalized inflammation

This is rarely seen beneath new complete dentures unless there is an unstable occlusion or obliteration of the freeway space. The correction of these conditions is not a practice emergency as such because either the denture has to be remade or at least the prosthetic teeth have to be removed and repositioned.

It might also be produced by a candida infection or very rarely by a tissue response to any free monomer remaining in the acrylic.

Management. A suspicion of an allergic reaction to the materials has to be confirmed by patch tests carried out under controlled conditions.

For management of a candida infection under complete dentures *see* Chapter 5, p. 50.

Localized bruising and ulceration on the denture – bearing mucosa

A localized sore spot on the denture bearing mucosa, can be caused by an occlusal interference or an unstable base.

Management. Identify the correct site by using pressure paste on the fit surface of the denture base. Instruct the patient to move the mandible into all excursions to identify any displacing occlusal interferences.

If a displacing interference is present, this must be marked with articulating paper and adjusted. Frequently the interference is related to the teeth immediately over the site of the sore spot.

The cause of sore areas in the denture bearing area of the palate may be difficult to identify and treat. They may be caused by occlusal imbalance, processing errors or, at worst, a faulty impression. The latter would require a total rebase.

A mandibular complete denture is always likely to move during mastication and sharp areas on the fit surface (where the impression material has flowed into a fold in the mucosa) may produce ulceration at that site. The fit surface must always be examined for processing errors, for example projections from the surface caused by tiny bubbles.

Localized bruising and ulceration related to the periphery

Usually this is due to over extension of the periphery of the denture base, and presents as a painful, erythematous or ulcerated mucosa adjacent to the over extended periphery. It is also likely to occur in the floor of the mouth in the region of the mylohyoid ridge.

Patients who have lost most of the alveolar bone in the mandible, present with pain and sometimes paraesthesia of the lower lip on that side. This might be due to pressure of the denture base directly on the mental nerve.

Management. Locate the site of an over extension of the denture base with pressure paste. Adjust and polish the base.

Bear in mind:

(i) Oedema from inflammation will itself cause ulceration. Any adjustment must be enough only to reduce the acute discomfort. Once the oedema has subsided the tissues may no longer impinge on the periphery of the denture base.

(ii) Ulceration beneath a complete denture can be the result of pressure caused by swelling related to underlying pathology, such as a retained root, an erupting tooth or a cystic lesion.

Palatal ulceration

Over extension of the posterior border may cause ulceration and discomfort during swallowing. If the posterior seal is too prominent, ulceration of the palate may result.

Management. The site of the over extension must be located and adjusted. If the base is extended too far posteriorly on to the soft palate, any adjustment which reduces the denture base at this site may remove the posterior seal. This must be replaced using self cure acrylic if retention of the prosthesis is to be restored.

If the site of the ulceration is at the junction between the hard and soft palate, the posterior seal must be reduced but not completely removed.

Cheek biting

This is commonly caused by an edge-to-edge occlusion between the buccal cusps of opposing posterior teeth.

Management. A horizontal overlap must be provided by rounding the buccal cusps of the mandibular posterior teeth. If the problem is a result of incorrect tooth position in the canine region, the upper canines have to be removed and repositioned with the tip inclined more palatally. Add acrylic to buccal surfaces.

FRACTURED COMPLETE DENTURE

Where a small part of the denture base has chipped away and is rough to the tongue or cheek use an acrylic bur to reshape the fractured margin and then polish it.

Where a large part of the denture is broken away or the base is fractured through, some laboratory assistance will be required. These fractures impair the retention and/or the appearance of the prosthesis.

Management

- Reassemble the various pieces of the fractured prosthesis, which may be stabilized one to the other using a cyanoacrylate cement. Great care has to be taken to ensure that the alignment of the fragments is correct and for this an assistant is essential.
- Block out the undercuts in the fit surface of the base and pour a plaster cast (not stone) into the fit surface of the prosthesis. Carefully remove the cast from the prosthesis and treat the surface of the cast with a separating medium. Cut out each fracture line and make space for a sufficient amount of self cure acrylic to be placed which will not only repair the fracture but be rigid enough not to fracture itself. Replace the prosthesis on the cast and paint monomer carefully into the freshly cut surfaces adjacent to the original fracture line. Run self cure acrylic resin into the repair area.
- If possible the acrylic should be allowed to cure under pressure and in hot water. This can be done by placing the repaired prosthesis on the cast in a pressure pot. If no such device is available it is prudent to place the repair in hot (not boiling) water to accelerate the curing process and remove some of the excess monomer.
- Remove excess material and polish the prosthesis.
- If the repaired prosthesis is not stable, an immediate provisional rebase may be carried out as a temporary measure (soft reline with rebase material). This procedure is not as straightforward as it may appear at first because of the occlusal problems which it invariably causes.

IMMEDIATE REPLACEMENT DENTURES

Problems associated with immediate replacement dentures may be divided into surgical and prosthodontic phases, although in practice these overlap.

Problems related to the surgical phase

Poor technique at the surgical phase may result in poorly contoured margins of the sockets or inadequate removal of an undercut from bony protuberances. These problems are of more importance when a labial flange is present on the denture than when the teeth are individually 'socketed'.

Management

- Before adjusting the denture, always ensure that the site of surgery is healing and that there is no evidence of a retained root or other foreign body which, if present, must be removed. Any sharp bony margin of a socket must be smoothed.
- Bleeding from the surgical site may be a complication although a prosthesis with a flange acts as a pressure pack. If bleeding is encountered, remove the prosthesis and wash it under running water. Identify the cause of the bleeding (*see* Chapter 4) and rectify. Replace the prosthesis in the mouth.

Problems related to the prosthodontic phase

Discomfort may arise from inadequacies in the surgical phase (eg. retained roots, sequestrae, sharp socket margins) or in the construction of the denture itself. Inspect the fit surface of the denture for irregularities. If there are none evident consider that, in the preparation of the cast, too much stone had been removed when assessing the form of the postoperative ridge. This will produce a denture which tends to bind on the bony margins and ulcerate the overlying mucosa.

When many natural teeth have been removed at one visit (usually anterior teeth), it is imperative that the denture is not removed for the first 24 hours post-operatively. The patient might not be able to reseat it in the mouth.

Management

- Relieve the fit surface of the prosthesis although this may reduce the stability of the base.
- Where a single tooth immediate replacement has been 'socketed', there is a danger that the projection of the artificial tooth into the tissue is too deep and may impinge on the ridge. Trim the acrylic at the neck of the tooth to allow room for pressure-free healing.
- Advise the patient to keep to a soft diet and prescribe analgesics such as paracetamol.

FRACTURES IN PARTIAL DENTURES

Loss of function of a clasp

The loss of retention of a partial denture may be due to a fractured clasp or to its having been bent out of shape. Before adjusting a clasp always warn the patient that it may fracture. If the clasp has fractured it will be necessary to replace it.

Management

- Make an impression of the denture in the mouth. Pour a cast with the denture in the impression. Form a new clasp around the abutment tooth on the cast and embed the retention tag into a channel cut in the existing acrylic of the prosthesis. Secure the new clasp with self cure acrylic.
- Sometimes the retention may be improved by the addition of self cure acrylic to the guide planes of the prosthesis. Add the acrylic to those areas which guide the prosthesis into position particularly around the crowns of the last standing abutment teeth. Insert and remove the prosthesis several times while the acrylic is setting. Place it in hot water. Trim away the excess when the material has set hard. Polish the addition.

Fracture of a major connector

If a major connector is bent or fractured a new prosthesis will have to be made. It may be possible to fabricate a temporary denture from the pieces of the old one until arrangements are made to make a replacement.

Immediate additions to partial dentures

It is sometimes necessary to add a tooth to a partial denture following an unexpected extraction.

Management

1. Shape a piece of tin foil over the extraction site in the mouth using a sprinkling of denture adhesive to hold it in place. Clean and key the replacement denture tooth and that part of the denture base which will receive it with a bur.

2. Apply self cure acrylic resin to the fit surface of the denture tooth and the keyed portion of the denture base. When the resin is about to set, place the denture in the mouth and position the denture tooth according to the occlusion and the appearance. Remove any excess acrylic and complete the final curing by placing the denture in a pressure flask.

3. Any further adjustments and additions may then be made before removing the tin foil. Shape the addition and polish it, ensuring that the occlusion is satisfactory.

13: Orthodontic Emergencies
A.J. Rodesano

Orthodontic emergencies are always related to patients wearing removable or fixed appliances.

REMOVABLE APPLIANCES

Breakages

Breakages can occur to

1. wire components
2. acrylic base.

Management

- Broken wire components. If the appliance is being worn without discomfort, ask the patient to continue wearing it until time is available for repair.

  When a broken wire component renders the appliance unwearable, it should be repaired as soon as possible. Broken springs will need to be replaced. Remove the remaining piece from the acrylic, and fashion a new one. Reattach it to the appliance using cold-cure acrylic. Fractured cribs or clasps can be soldered and replaced if necessary at a later date.
- Broken acrylic bases. Invariably these require a major repair. If the break is clean, replace the appliance in the mouth, and take an overall impression, for model construction, with the appliance *in situ*. Once located in the plaster, remove acrylic from either side of the fracture line within the appliance and repair using cold-cure acrylic, polymerizing under pressure. Sometimes it is possible, where there is a clean break and no evidence of distortion, to relocate the fragments and to hold them with sticky wax or cyanoacylate glue. The appliance may be located in plaster and processed as above. Where there is evidence of distortion, take an impression of the mouth prior to the repair, without the appliance *in situ*. Reconstruct the appliance as necessary.

Disorted wire components

Wire components which are impinging upon soft tissues should be reshaped or removed as appropriate.

II FIXED APPLIANCES

    (a)   Loose bands
    (b)   Loose direct bonded or welded attachments
    (c)   Fractured or displaced wires
    (d)   Loose ligatures.

Management

- *Loose bands.* Loose bands may be displaced totally and interfere with mastication or speech, or partially displaced and irritate the marginal gingivae. They may give rise to ulceration, haemorrhage, oedema or gingival recession. Loss of cement seal and subsequent plaque deposition may lead to decalcification. Where instrumentation is available, remove the loose or damaged bands. After cleaning drying and reshaping, check them for fit. Prepare the tooth or teeth with pumice and dry thoroughly, and recement the band. When arch wires are in the way, resite them and religature as appropriate.

  Where suitable instrumentation is unavailable, remove the bands, reshape the ends of the arch wire with pliers to render them atraumatic, and instruct the patient to contact the orthodontist as soon as possible.

- *Loose attachments.* Loose direct bonded attachments seldom present as an emergency unless they are carrying the end of an arch wire. If matching attachments and bonding materials are not available, remove the displaced units and render the arch wire safe. If tube attachments carrying the ends of an arch wire become detached, reshape the wire to prevent damage to the adjacent soft tissues. Remove welded attachments which have become loosened from the bands with pliers. The bands may be left in situ until time is available for their removal and replacement.

  An individual intra-arch band which loses attachment from a tooth should be fixed loosely to the arch wire, with a ligature around the cervical margin. This prevents the tooth moving out of the control of the arch wire.

- *Fractured or displaced wires.* Fractured, distorted or displaced wires or ligatures may impinge on soft tissue and cause irritation and ulceration. If possible, replace them, or reshape them with pliers to relieve trauma. Where arch wires are embedded in soft tissue, as may occur with multi-looped wires, apply local anaesthetic paste or infiltrate local anaesthetic, and divide the enclosing mucosa to release the wire. After seven to ten days, when oedema has settled and the mucosa healed, the arch wire may be replaced clear of the mucosa.
- *Loose ligatures.* Loose ligatures may be tightened or replaced.

Pain

Following appliance fixation or adjustment, pain may be expected. Patients should be reassured that slight discomfort is normal for the first 48 hours. Should it be troublesome, prescribe aspirin or paracetamol.

External trauma

Patients wearing fixed or removable appliances may be involved in traumatic incidents and pieces of the appliances may be lost or displaced, and parts may be unaccounted for. Examine the patient's mouth with great care and, if parts of the appliance are missing, refer the patient to the Accident and Emergency Department of the local hospital. Radiographs may be required of the chest and abdomen. The patient's orthodontist should be contacted as soon as practicable.

14:   Misadventures in the Surgery

IATROGENIC TRAUMA — TRAUMA INFLICTED BY THE OPERATOR OR ASSISTANT

Accidents will happen to the most careful operator in the best-organized of practices. It is essential however to provide, for the patients and the staff, a safe working environment and sound working methods. Where accidents do occur, the law requires the practitioner to behave as any reasonable individual would, having received a similar training and being in similar circumstances.

1. Record the events in the notes, in your own hand — the circumstances of the injury, what was done, what was said and how it was repaired. This should be done as soon as possible after the event is under control.
2. Always and immediately inform your medical defence organization.
3. If there is doubt in your mind as to whether you are competent to repair the damage, for example a laceration, consult with a colleague and/or refer to hospital.

Lacerations

The treatment should be similar to that provided to a patient traumatized by a third party, *see* Chapter 3, p. 28.

The fractured jaw

Except for the straightforward extraction, all teeth should have a radiograph to show the complete root formation before extraction is attempted. *All wisdom teeth must have a pre-extraction radiograph, the lower ones preferably to include the lower border of the mandible.*

During the removal of any tooth, if the operator or the patient suspects that a fracture of the jaw may have occurred, a radiograph must be taken immediately, before the extraction is completed. If the tooth is loose, complete the extraction *with great care*, and examine the root for fracture and retained elements. Examine the alveolar bone and, if there is any suspicion that there might be a fracture, take a radiograph to show detail of the bone adjacent and apical to the socket. If the mandible is involved, the lower border must be visible on the film.

The fractured alveolar process

The alveolar process may fracture and remain adherent to the tooth in any part of the mouth, with the anterior region the most commonly affected. Usually the labial plate only is involved. The alveolar process supporting adjacent teeth may fracture and, where the maxillary molar teeth are being extracted, such fractures may involve the floor of the antrum. *Where adjacent maxillary molar teeth require extraction, always commence with the most posterior tooth.*

If a fractured alveolar process is suspected:

1. Stop the extraction and inspect the tooth and adjacent tissues.
2. If a segment of the alveolus appears to be moving with the tooth, ascertain if one or both plates are involved. If a single plate, dissect it free of the mucosa and suture the wound. If a segment of the alveolar process appears to be moving, either:
   (a) Abandon the extraction. Wait three or four weeks, and complete it using a surgical approach.
   (b) Splint the tooth if necessary, using figure-of-eight wiring to the adjacent teeth, or by placing a vacuum-formed polycarbonate overlay on the teeth.
   (c) Suture any lacerations in the mucoperiosteum.
   (d) Prescribe antibiotics — ampicillin or erythromycin 250 mg four times a day for five days.
   or
   (a) Raise buccal and lingual/palatal flaps
   (b) Gutter around the tooth and roots with a bur, attempting to conserve as much alveolar bone as possible.
   (c) Remove the tooth.
   (d) Inspect the wound and remove any bone which is likely to have lost its blood supply.
   (e) Suture the wound to appose the mucosa as far as possible over the socket.
   (f) If an oro antral fistula is suspected proceed as below (page 112).
   (g) Prescribe antibiotics — ampicillin or erythromycin 250 mg four times a day for five days.

The fractured mandible

If a fractured mandible is suspected during an extraction

1. Stop the procedure.
2. Grasp the mandible each side of the tooth being extracted and attempt to 'spring' the fracture. If there is a suspicion of movement and/or the patient complains of pain at the site of the extraction a fracture is likely. Note that pain may be experienced when a fracture is manipulated, even when a successful inferior alveolar injection has been administered.
3. Take a radiograph to show bone detail, apical to the tooth and including the lower border of the mandible.
4. If a fracture is identified or suspected, *tell the patient*, and refer to hospital by telephone.
5. Ensure that the patient can be transported to hospital. The patient should not drive. If necessary, provide a taxi at your own expense. Do not drive the patient to hospital in your own car unless it is insured for this eventuality.
6. A temporary splinting of the mandible by bandage or eyelet wires may be helpful.
7. Record the events in detail in your own hand in the notes. Ensure that all radiographs are conserved.

Oro-antral fistula

This may occur during the extraction of any of the upper molar teeth. A fistula rarely occurs as far forward as the first premolar. If there is a suspicion that an oro–antral fistula may have been created during an extraction, inspect the wound using an aspirator and listen for the typical deep resonance. Be wary about inserting an instrument into the wound. Many small fistulae heal without treatment. If a fistula is suspected:

1. Inform the patient.
2. If the socket is small and undamaged, no further local treatment is required. If the socket is wide and expanded, compress the alveolus digitally, and insert a mattress suture.
3. Advise the patient not to blow the nose for a week, explaining the reasons for this.
4. If the tooth or its gingivae were infected prior to the extraction, prescribe antibiotics (ampicillin or tetracycline, 250 mg four times a day for five days).

If there is a fracture of the alveolus which might lead to an oro-antral fistula, proceed as follows:

1. Raise a broad-based buccal flap and inspect the alveolar bone as the tooth is moved.
2. Raise a palatal flap if the buccal mucosa appears to be adherent to the alveolar bone or if it is lacerated.
3. Create a gutter in the bone around the roots of the tooth using a fissure bur, attempting to conserve as much bone as possible.
4. Remove the tooth.
5. Inspect the wound carefully for an oro-antral fistula and remove all unattached bone fragments.
6. Get the patient to blow *gently* against an occluded nasal airway, inspecting the socket for the egress of air or bulging antral mucosa.
7. Advance the buccal flap by incising the periosteum horizontally high in the base of the mucoperiosteal flap, and above the mucosal reflection in the sulcus. The advancement should continue until the flap lies passively covering the socket.
8. Remove damaged or devitalized mucosa from the edges of the flaps. On the palatal side, the mucosa should be trimmed back until not less than a millimeter of palatal bone is exposed on which to rest the flap. Very rarely, it is impossible to achieve this due to excessive loss of bone. The prognosis for a successful closure is very much reduced if the buccal flap is not closed over the bone.
9. Occasionally, it is necessary to remove an adjacent tooth where its root is exposed into the fistula, with no bone covering it. Failure to do so will result in a breakdown of the suture line and the re-establishment of an oro-antral fistula.
10. Insert vertical mattress sutures to evert the edges of the flap, and close the wound with interrupted sutures. Use only the minimum number of sutures to achieve this. The blood supply to the edges of the flap will be compromised if too many are used.
11. Prescribe antibiotics (ampicillin or tetracycline as above) and a nasal decongestant, 0.1% Otrivine.
12. Inform the patient that the nose must not be blown for one week in the first instance, explaining the reasons for this.
13. See the patient to remove the sutures and check the wound at one week.
14. Advise the patient that nose blowing may need to be abandoned

for a further week or done gently — according to the state of healing of the wound.
15. A further check-up at three months is advisable, taking a history for possible sinus symptoms.

Important: In all cases where an oro-antral fistula is suspected, full explanations must be given to the patient and good records kept in the notes. Post-extraction radiographs may be helpful and should be preserved carefully.

If you do not feel competent to repair the oro-antral fistula as described above, immediately refer to a department of oral surgery by telephone.

Broken rotary instrument

All instruments used in dental practise are capable of breaking or coming apart. Most misadventures are unexpected and inadvertent. It is important to follow a set procedure when such misadventures do occur.

1. Stop the procedure.
2. Instruct the patient and your assistant to remain still. Keep the aspirator tip away from the presumed site of the missing fragment.
3. Inspect the remains of the instrument and make an estimate as to the size and shape of the retained part.
4. Move the patient and illumination to the optimum position.
5. Search methodically for the broken piece. If, for example, a bur has broken during an oral surgical procedure, search in the area in which the intact bur was last seen. Search the adjacent soft tissues, then the sulci and pouches into which the piece may have fallen. Finally search the oro-pharynx as well as possible, or the throat pack, if used. If these searches prove unavailing then proceed to (6).
6. Change the aspirator bottle, and irrigate the aspirator with generous quantities of water. Where there is no aspirator bottle, replace the filter in the machine, and run through copious quantities of water. Sift through the 'old' filter or bottle, keeping all solid objects.
7. Search the floor, the drapes and bib, and the clothing of the patient, of the operator and of the assistant. As appropriate, search under the surgery furniture, and under closed doors.

8. Take intra-oral radiographs in the first instance, of the operation site. If the object remains unidentified, take a larger radiograph such as an orthopantomogram or lateral oblique. If the object still is not located, refer to hospital for a chest and/or abdominal radiograph.
9. Keep the patient informed at all times as to what has happened and explain the reasons for the steps you are taking.
10. Record in detail, in your own hand in the patient's notes, the events as they occurred, and the efforts you made to find the broken or lost piece. If it had been necessary to refer the patient to hospital, record the time that you telephoned the hospital and the name of the person to whom you spoke. This should be done as soon as the emergency is over.

In emergency situations, it is inappropriate to refer the patient to hospital by letter alone. Telephone to inform the consultant concerned and arrange for the patient to be seen, and send the patient with a detailed letter of referral.

Bear in mind: in oral surgical procedures, sometimes it is better to continue the operation, if the operator is convinced that the instrument remains in the wound. It may be necessary to use further burs to give vision or access to the place where the broken instrument may have lodged.

Broken needle or small foreign body in soft tissues

Now that all needles are disposable and used only once, fractured needles are rare. Suturing needles fracture more commonly, but usually this occurs in a needle that has already been distorted. Therefore, *never straighten a bent needle*; discard it, and proceed with a new one. Identifying the broken suturing needle requires a procedure identical with that for the broken oral surgical instrument (*see* above). The broken injection needle usually is identified at the time of the injection and the procedure should be as follows:

1. Inform the patient, and request him or her not to move.
2. *Without moving your eyes from the site of the injection*, ask your assistant for a fibre-tipped pen or fountain pen (not a ball-point), to mark the position of the needle entry. Alternatively, ask your assistant for a second charged syringe, inject a small 'bubble' of local anaesthetic close to the first injection site, and mark the position with a small incision with a scalpel blade.

3. Infiltrate more local anaesthetic solution beneath your mark, as symmetrically as possible, and wait a few minutes. Use sufficient solution only to produce anaesthesia; the more you use, the more distortion there will be of the tissues.

4. Prepare a full set of instruments as for a minor oral surgical procedure. If it is your practice not to have a set, refer to hospital. Do not try to find the foreign body if you have inadequate instrumentation.

5. Incise the mucosa superficially and widely (about 2 cm). Use blunt dissection systematically from a point slightly anterior to the anticipated site of the retained needle. This allows a retractor to be inserted in front of the fragment, and the search will be posteriorly to it.

6. Blunt dissection, spreading rounded (not pointed) scissors or a Spencer Wells forcep progressively through the tissues, will identify most pieces. Metal objects deep in soft tissue may be localized by exploration with a blunt metal instrument. A small fragment is easier to identify with a fine delicate instrument. Never hesitate to use a gloved finger as the exploring tool — it is probably the best of the lot! Seeing the object, so that it may be grasped and removed, will be far more difficult.

7. If the above fails to identify the position of the fragment within a few minutes, take radiographs. Two will be required, from different angles, with a 90° difference being the ideal. It is helpful to insert two identifiable radio-opaque objects (a suture needle and a root canal reamer suitably secured with floss, for example) into the tissues in close vicinity to the anticipated position of the lost fragment, prior to taking the radiograph. *Leave these objects in position*, develop the film and, by parallax effects, the position of the fragment will be located.

8. If the needle fractures while giving an inferior alveolar block, all the above advice applies *only* if it is anticipated that the remains of the needle lie just beneath the mucosa.

9. The most successful attempt to find a buried metal object is the first. If you are unsure about your abilities, refer to hospital straight away by telephone, *but not before applying a surface marking as described above*. Give the patient a letter for the hospital, containing a detailed description of the events, and enclose the remaining fragment to take with them. Arrange for a taxi to take the patient to hospital, perhaps at your own expense, resisting the temptation to drive the patient there in your own car unless you car insurance covers you for this.

10. Record the events in your own hand in the patient's notes. The entry should include a description of the episode and the procedures you initiated. It should be done as soon after the event as possible.

Falls, blows, etc.

Should a patient or member of staff fall on your premises or suffer a blow to the person, you should behave as any reasonable person would if the similar events occurred in your own home. If there is the possibility that the patient might feel that the damage had occurred as a result of their having dental treatment, additional precautions should be taken. For example, a local anaesthetic may have been given, and the patient might feel that, in some way, this had contributed to the fall.

1. Comfort the patient.
2. Where reasonable, examine the patient's injury and/or damage to the patient's property.
3. Where there is cause for suspicion of internal injuries (e.g. a fractured bone), refer to the accident and emergency department at the local hospital. Arrange transport, or summon an ambulance. Do not take the patient in your own car, unless you are insured to do so.
4. Record the events in the patient's notes. If the patient fails to take your advice, record this in the notes too.
5. The most effective way to abort a suit for damages is to reassure the patient repeatedly that all the necessary steps are being taken.

If any of the above should occur on public property, such as a hospital or community clinic, complete an accident form. Have you checked your third party insurance recently to ensure that you are covered adequately?

Complications of inferior alveolar block injections

It is not infrequent that trismus follows an inferior alveolar injection. The trismus may be rapid in onset, developing soon after normal sensation returns to the anaesthetized area, or it may develop more slowly over two to three days. While the mechanism is unknown, it is assumed that the needle on its passage to the inferior alveolar nerve, causes bleeding into or adjacent to the medial pterygoid muscle. The subsequent inflammation promotes trismus.

Management

1. Reassurance and explanation, to allay the patient's understand-able fears. Specifically, it is important to stress that it is a fairly common phenomenon, that it will resolve with time, and that it is not caused by infection.
2. Advise resting the jaw for a week, with no attempt to force opening of the mouth. This allows any inflammation to subside. Many will recover in this time. For those who do not:
3. Advise progressive exercise. This may be done passively with the patient opening the mouth against the resistance of the trismus, measuring the opening by the number of fingers which can be inserted between the incisor teeth.

   A more active method is to use wooden tongue depressors (spatulas). Advise the patient to stack a number of the spatulas and lay them across the mouth, holding them between the canines and premolars of the opposing jaws in a posture similar to that of a dog holding a bone. When the apparent maximum number is reached, further ones may be added by separating two of the spatulas and inserting another into the gap so created. This should be continued progressively until trismus and pain permit no further spatulas to be fitted during that session. The exercise should be done over a ten minute period, night and morning. Advise the patient that, although it hurts to do this, it will do no harm. The exercise should be repeated each day with the attempt to add a further spatula each night, and to achieve the same number the next morning. Within a few days, normal opening usually is achieved.
4. If the above fails, or the patient appears to be dissatisfied, refer to the local oral surgery unit with a request for the patient to be seen soon. A second opinion, with the consultant offering similar reassurance and treatment, will satisfy the patient who may have felt that the condition could have been the result of malpractice.

Sustained anaesthesia, hypoaesthesia, dysaesthesia

Rarely, the inferior alveolar injection may be inserted into the nerve trunk itself. The consequence may be temporary nerve damage leading to change in sensation in the distribution of that nerve.

Management. Explanation and reassurance may be required in abundance. If there is fear of possible medicolegal consequencies, refer to hospital for urgent consultation. This may reduce patient anxiety. There is no active treatment.

Bear in mind: It is possible that the nerve block itself may not be to blame. Could your treatment to the anaesthetized area be the cause — for example, did you damage the inferior alveolar nerve when you elevated the third molar, or did your root canal filling pass through the apex of the second premolar and enter the inferior dental canal?

15:   Emergency Hospital Management of Facial Pain

The hospital practitioner is advised to refer to Chapter 1, for details of each condition. Management which could be carried out by dental practitioners in their practice will be found there. Such treatment may be appropriate to the hospital practitioner too, depending upon the circumstances of each individual case.

I   UNILATERAL SHARP PAIN

Paroxysmal trigeminal and glossopharyngeal neuralgia

In the acute phase, this condition may be treated as follows:

1. Local anaesthetics

As stated in Chapter 1, local anaesthetic solution, preferably bupivacaine, may be injected around the peripheral nerve which serves as the trigger area. This is also helpful for diagnosis. If the trigger is abolished, the diagnosis is confirmed. The anaesthesia produced will give the patient relief of pain for up to 12 hours using bupivacaine. Occasionally, the relief may extend to weeks or months. In most cases however, it is wise to commence drug therapy as follows, seeing the patient at short regular intervals to adjust the dose until the pain is controlled.

2. Carbamazepine

Start at 100 mg three times a day and increase by 100 mg every three days in divided doses until control is achieved or side effects of dizziness and/or drowsiness prevent further increase. The maximum dose is 1200 mg. Early side effects may be avoided by commencing with 50 mg three times a day increasing by 50 mg per day for three to four days.

119

3. Phenytoin

Where there are early side effects or incomplete control with carbamazepine, phenytoin starting with a dose of 100 mg twice per day, and increasing slowly to a maximum of 600 mg in divided doses if necessary. Baclofen and sodium valproate are alternatives.

4. Cryotherapy

This involves freezing the peripheral nerve as it is exiting the foramen usually under local analgesia. It is helpful in the emergency situation, where a patient with established trigeminal neuralgia has severe paroxysms of pain no longer controlled by drug therapy at maximum tolerated doses. This should be done only after discussion with a consultant.

II UNILATERAL DULL PAIN

TM joint dysfunction

The acute phase of TM joint dysfunction can be most painful and distressing. It can follow direct violence, such as a blow to the joint, or indirect violence from a blow to the chin. Where there is a history of violence, radiographs should be taken to exclude a fracture. Often, it arises following a wide yawn, eating a hard bolus of food, or simply shouting. In these situations, it can be assumed that the pain is arising as a result of damage to the soft tissues of the joint. Examination may reveal an effusion, and a deranged occlusion with the teeth on the affected side not meeting fully – a lateral open bite. There will be trismus, but this should not be confused with the trismus arising from muscle hyperactivity alone where the joint will exhibit little or no tenderness.

Less frequently, and more commonly following TMJ surgery, the patient may complain of severe pain reminiscent of cramp, felt deep to the joint, for as long as 10 minutes. It may be triggered by joint movement, particularly in the cold. It is assumed that this is due to spasm of the lateral pterygoid muscle. The pain is temporarily incapacitating.

Treatment

When there is a history of trauma, exclude a fracture of the condylar neck before initiating treatment, by taking a radiograph, preferably using a panoramic X-ray machine.

1. Local anaesthetic — to relieve severe acute pain arising from the joint itself, an auriculotemporal block using bupivacaine will relieve the pain rapidly and produce anasthaesia for up to 10 hours. When sensation returns, generally the pain will be less than previously. The hypodermic needle is inserted immediately behind the posterior border of the condylar neck about 1 cm inferior to the joint, with the needle directed medially and forward so that the solution is deposited to the medial side of the condylar neck. About 2 ml are used; more than this will be certain to produce temporary facial paralysis. Precautions should be taken to protect the eye where the blink reflex is slow or lost.

2. Analgesics — non-steroidal anti-inflammatory drugs (NSAIDS) may be very helpful. The most effective and safest is ibuprofen 400–600 mg six hourly. This not only produces pain relief but

actively reduces inflammation. It should be continued for a week and the patient reviewed. Intra-articular steroid injections should *not* be used, as they may cause irreversible damage to the articulation, and offer little additional benefit. Lesser discomfort may be controlled by aspirin and paracetamol preparations, or similar peripherally-acting analgesics. Narcotics should be avoided, because of side effects in the ambulant patient.

3.   Muscle relaxants — acute cramp-like pains of muscle spasm, particularly after surgery, are well controlled by baclofen 5–10 mg three times a day. Seldom is this required for more than two weeks. Where there is a large element of masticatory muscle tenderness, a tricyclic drug such as dothiepin should be commenced at a dose of 75 mg at night, increasing to 150 mg if necessary, in the knowledge that it will not have immediate effect but will begin to act only after a few days. Where there is a large element of anxiety, a sedative such as fluphenazine may be added. A useful combination preparation containing nortryptiline 30 mg and fluphenazine hydrochloride 1.5 mg is Motipress, taken at night.

Herpes zoster (shingles)

In the acute phase, where the second and third divisions of the trigeminal nerve are involved, this can be confused with toothache; indeed, it is not uncommon for the patient to be referred to hospital after extractions have been carried out, with apparent complications of that extraction. The developing vescicles are mistaken for infection spreading from the sockets, or even acute ulcerative gingivitis. Frequently, particularly if the patient is elderly, the pain may be sufficiently severe to make admission necessary for pain control and maintenance of fluid balance. If admission is contemplated, consider putting the patient in an isolation ward during the vesicular stage.

Treatment

- Pain relief — aspirin or paracetamol compounds, or ibuprofen are usually sufficient. Aspirin and papaveretum tablets, two to four hourly, are a little stronger. If pain is severe, narcotics may have to be considered. Dextromoramide 5–10 mg four to six hourly orally may be helpful. Buprenorphine should be avoided in the elderly, because of its side effects.
- Secondary infection — chlorhexidine mouth wash will reduce the extent of secondary infection. Tetracycline mouthbath alone, or

tetracycline and amphotericin syrup would be advisable in the more severe case. If there is evidence of spreading systemic infection, with increasing pyrexia, and cervical lymphadenopathy, systemic broad spectrum antibiotics become necessary, for example, amoxycillin 250–500 mg three times per day for five days.

- General management — the patient may become debilitated through insufficient fluid and calorie intake. It may be necessary to set up an intravenous drip to restore fluid balance. Parenteral feeding is not necessary. To assist the patient to eat and drink, benzydamine hydrochloride (Difflam) oral rinse prior to food is helpful.
- Depression frequently accompanies shingles and may be present early in the disease. It may be profound and many elderly patients become suicidal. An antidepressant such as amitryptiline, 25–50 mg daily, together with sodium valproate 200 mg three times per day may be helpful, both in controlling pain and mood, but also to reduce the chance of severe post-herpetic neuralgia. In the elderly male, avoid tricyclic drugs where there is a history of prostatism. In established cases of post herpetic neuralgia similar doses of psychotropic drugs are helpful. EMLA cream applied to the affected division can give the patient some relief.

Periodic migrainous neuralgia

This is a form of migraine, but the mechanism is not understood. In part it is due to anxiety — the very fear that an attack is imminent may be sufficient to begin an attack. There may be a premonition that the pain is about to arise which is different for each individual, and may vary from a visual disturbance, to an odour or a particular facial sensation.

Treatment

- Ergotamine preparations are beneficial, but rapid absorption is essential. Thus preparations that are absorbed in the gut are inappropriate. Rapid release and absorption preparations such as Lingraine (ergotamine tartrate 2 mg), which is dissolved under the tongue, or medihaler-ergotamine (ergotamine tartrate 360 μg as an aerosol oral inhaler), are useful. The patient should be told that the maximum permissible use for the tablets is two daily or six weekly and, for the inhalations, six daily and 15 weekly. This avoids the potential complication of peripheral vascular disease.
- The essential factor for the successful treatment of periodic

migrainous neuralgia is that the rapid release preparations should be used *as soon as the patient has the premonition that the attack is about to occur.*

- For those who get their attacks at times when it is impossible to use the above preparations, for instance when they are woken from sleep with the pain, seratonine antagonists should be prescribed. Methysergide is probably the most effective at a dose of 1 mg three times a day, prescribed for three week periods with a week-free period. This avoids the potentially dangerous complications of retroperitoneal fibrosis. Pizotifen 500 μg three times a day is a useful alternative. Some physicians find propranolol, 40 mg three times a day, useful but the side effects can be a undesirable.

- A particular feature of periodic migrainous neuralgia is that it is characterized by exacerbations and remissions. The patients live in fear of an attack and, as anxiety can provoke an attack, it can become self-perpetuating. When a treatment is found which prevents an attack, the patient becomes more confident, and an exacerbation may remit; the patient has the reassurance of the successful ergot preparation in the pocket, and finds that it is not necessary to take it.

Cranial arteritis

Cranial arteritis needs speedy management. With a history of pain described in Chapter 1, it is important to consider the diagnosis, particularly in the elderly patient. It is always expedient to attempt to elicit tenderness over the superficial temporal artery, but this is not a reliable sign. If it is tender, an arterial biopsy is easy to perform under local analgesia and should be done immediately. However, a more important test is the erythrocyte sedimentation rate (ESR), and the result is ready in an hour. The patient should wait for the result. If the ESR is raised, and there is no other likely cause, treatment must start at the first visit.

Treatment

- Prescribe prednisolone, 60 mg per day in divided doses. If the patient has conditions such as peptic ulceration, which might be aggravated by systemic steroids, appropriate measures should be taken under the direction of a physician. Prednisolone may be reduced as the ESR and symptoms reduce, until a small maintenance dose is achieved. The patient should be referred to a physician for further management.

III BILATERAL DULL PAIN

Sinusitis

Where sinusitis is suspected, with tenderness to palpation over the maxillary sinuses and sometimes the frontal sinuses, occipito-mental radiographs should be taken to confirm the diagnosis. If the problem is acute-on-chronic, the patient should be referred to an otolaryngologist. Other causes, such as spread from a dental abscess or an oro-antral fistula, must be excluded.

Treatment

- *Analgesics*: aspirin and paracetamol preparations usually suffice. Ibuprofen is a useful alternative.
- *Antibiotics*: broad spectrum antibiotics such as tetracycline or ampicillin, 250 mg four times a day are best, prescribed for not less than five days.
- *Nasal decongestants*: (Otrivine) 0.1% as nasal drops or spray, is effective for up to eight hours and causes little nasal discomfort. Steam inhalations with *Tinc. Benz. Co.* or Karvol added, are recommended. These serve to moisten the nasal passages, freeing them of encrusted material.
- *Antral washouts*: in obstinate sinusitis, antral washouts are required. This should be done in consultation with a department of otolaryngology

Atypical facial pain

This diagnosis should only be made after excluding pathology. Thus careful investigation must be included in the initial consultation. Seldom is the pain severe enough for the situation to be considered an emergency. Occasionally, patients present in pain, having had many ineffectual treatments, and will be anxious, even demanding, for effective treatment to begin.

Treatment

After exclusion of genuine pathology, foremost must be the reassurance of the patient. Where depression is predominant, tricyclic drugs at moderate dosage are generally successful (dothiepin 50–75 mg at night). If anxiety is associated with the depression, sedation may be added (a useful combination drug is Motipress – nortriptyline 25 mg, flufenazine 1 mg).

Atypical odontalgia

In this condition, the patient will be referred to hospital in acute pain. It is likely that the referring practitioner will have been to great lengths to investigate all possible dental causes of that pain and, over the past weeks a number of teeth may have been removed and pulps extirpated, with no apparent relief of symptoms. The patient will require the taking of a careful history and examination to exclude all other possible causes of the pain. Once the diagnosis is made, as has been stated in Chapter 1, *it is vital that all further dental treatment should be discontinued.*

Treatment

- The treatment to control atypical odontalgia can be successful only if the patient has confidence in the diagnosis. It is important therefore, that a senior and experienced clinician explains the condition and prescribes the treatment to promote that confidence. Time spent in explanation at the first consultation is well worthwhile. Unfortunately, the many attempts by the dental practitioner to alleviate the pain may have resulted in a number of inadequate root fillings or incomplete treatments. Any of these may give rise to pain too. Despite this, no further dental treatment should be given until the atypical odontalgia is under control.

- Dothiepin, beginning at a dose of 50 mg at night is effective, but this should be increased by 25 mg every three days, up to a maximum of 150 mg, until the pain is controlled. If the patient is extremely anxious or agitated, a sedative may be added. A useful combination preparation in this respect is Motipress (nortryptiline 25 mg. and fluphenazine 1 mg).

- Analgesics, such as ibuprofen may be added 400–600 mg six hourly. Sometimes it is necessary to add antibiotics such as amoxicillin 250 mg or metronidazole 200 mg three times per day, where periapical infections from inadequate root fillings for example, may be contributing to the discomfort.

Tumours

Where the symptoms and signs do not fulfil the criteria of any of the well-known conditions, or have abnormal features, always be suspicious that there could be a tumour causing the pain. For instance, tumours of the eighth cranial nerve — acoustic neuromas —

are notorious for mimicking other pathology. In the early stages of presentation, such tumours may cause transitory sharp or dull pains in the trigeminal distribution, always restricted to one side of the face. When a tumour is suspected as being the cause of facial pain, it is prudent to test for reduced sensation and motor loss in the distribution of all cranial nerves.

Dull pains may arise from spread of malignant tumours from the naso-pharynx or maxillary antrum into the trigeminal and other cranial nerves, as they leave the base of the skull. There may be diminished or absent sensation over parts of the face.

Management

1. *Naso-endoscopy.* The naso-endoscope is a most valuable tool in the diagnosis of nasopharyngeal tumours when the clinician is experienced in its use.
2. *Radiography.* Radiographs may be helpful in revealing certain tumours. A lateral view of the postnasal space, and an occipito-mental of the sinuses, may show a space-occupying lesion. Computed tomography (CT) or magnetic resonance imaging (MRI), are the most valuable investigations of all, and where there is sufficient indication, one of these scans should be arranged at the time of the emergency presentation, together with a chest X-ray to exclude metastases.

   Where possible, a biopsy should be taken, and sent to the histology laboratory in formol saline.
3. *Fine needle aspirate.* If an abnormal swelling is apparent, fine-needle aspiration may be very helpful. Take a large injection needle on a 2 ml syringe and pierce the swelling. Initial aspirate may reveal pus which can be sent on to the bacteriology laboratory for identification of the organism and antibacterial sensitivities. If no apparent aspirate is made, resposition the needle a few times, aspirating in each new position. Withdraw the needle, remove the syringe from the needle, and fill the syringe with air. Take two microscope slides, fit the needle back on to the syringe, and expel the contents of the needle on to one of the slides. Spread the aspirate thinly by compressing it with the second slide. Part the slides, leave one to dry in air, and spray the second with the fixative (the fixative used for cervical smears is ideal). From the smear, a skilled exfoliative cytologist may be able to make useful tentative diagnosis.

16: Emergency Management of Acute Swellings in Hospital

I INFLAMMATORY SWELLINGS

1. Make a diagnosis — *see* Chapter 2. If the abscess is thought to be periapical,
2. Take the patient's temperature.
3. If the patient is apyrexial, or has only a small pyrexia (less than 38°C)

    (a) Assess whether there is pus present. If a periapical collection may be forming, ream through the root canal of the affected tooth and establish drainage. If you feel that there is unlikely to be pus present, or access would be difficult:

    (b) Give antibiotics. Most oro-facial infections are caused by organisms sensitive to the penicillins (streptococci) or metronidazole (bacteroides), or both. If the patient is not sensitive to penicillin, give penicillin V or ampicillin 250 mg four times a day for five days. Alternatively, metronidazole 200 mg three times a day is satisfactory, especially if the patient is penicillin sensitive. Other alternatives are Cephradine 250 mg three times a day (but not where the patient has a history of severe penicillin sensitivity) or Erythromycin 250 mg four times a day.

    (c) If the patient is worse at 24 hours, or no better at 48 hours, *double the dose* of the antibiotic already prescribed. Examine the patient again at 48 hours without fail. Then:

    (d) If the patient has a pyrexia which is increasing, proceed as in (4) below.

    (e) If the infection is settling, make arrangements to eradicate the cause — remove the tooth, arrange for root canal filling etc.

4. If the patient is pyrexial, over 38°C:

    (a) Identify the location of the pus. If you feel that there is really no collection, prescribe antibiotics as above, but at double the dose. Metronidazole may be given in suppository form, 1G three times a day. If you feel that it is safe to send the patient home, *see them every 24 hours until the infection has subsided.*

Admit to hospital if there are symptoms of dysphagia, or the tongue is raised.

If there is a collection of pus but it is superficial, find the point of maximum fluctuation, use topical anaesthesia and incise. Ethyl chloride spray or topical lignocaine paste may be sufficient on the oral mucous membranes. Injected local anaesthetic solutions should only be used well away from the infected area. Occasionally, it is satisfactory and safe to raise a small 'blister' of local anaesthetic over the abscess and then to incise through it. *Never* infiltrate.

(b) If a collection of pus can be identified, *or you think that pus may be present,* admit the patient to hospital and arrange to incise and drain that day under general anaesthesia.

If you are unsure, if the temperature is rising, if there are signs of toxicity (headache, rigors, dizziness, nausea), *admit the patient to hospital.*

(c) Arrange for a full blood count, and take any additional radiographs to identify the cause and spread of the infection. Where the abscess is clear of hard tissues, the site and size may be estimated with the help of ultrasound. Very occasionally, CT scans may be required for instance, to assess whether the para-pharyngeal spaces are involved.

(d) Incise the abscess. Incise to produce dependent drainage. Usually this means incising extra-orally, choosing a site close to the abscess, but at a lower level, assuming that the patient will be nursed in an upright position postoperatively. If the patient is likely to have to lie in bed for a few days postoperatively, choose the site of your incision accordingly.

Make your incision large enough to insert a little finger into the abscess cavity. This will enable you to explore the cavity fully and to break down any loculi which have formed. Occasionally, as in the case of a child, the incision may be smaller, but the cavity *must* be explored with an instrument such as Hilton's forceps. Where there is trismus, it indicates usually that pus has developed in relation to the masseter and/or medial pterygoid. Explore on both sides of the mandible in relation to these muscles, particularly medially.

(e)   Drain. All abscess cavities require at least one drain. In superficial cavities in mobile tissue, a Penrose soft drain is sufficient. In larger, deeper cavities, use a corrugated drain. If the cavity straddles a structure such as the body of the mandible, use two drains, each sutured to the skin and identifiable individually.

(f)   Send the pus for bacteriological studies and ask for sensitivities. Tell the bacteriologist what antibiotics the patient has already been on. If actinomycosis is suspected, send as much of the pus as possible for centrifuging so that the 'ray fungus' may be identified.

(g)   Avoid giving antibiotics until the sensitivities are known. Where the patient is very unwell, set up a drip. This may be used to give bolus injections of antibiotic intravenously later, as well as restoring fluid balance. *Remember, pyrexic patients rapidly become dehydrated.*

(h)   Dress the wound with generous amounts of soft dressings. These should be changed at 12 hourly intervals. If the change of dressing cannot be witnessed, ask the nursing staff to keep the dressing for you to see. The amount of discharge on the dressing gives a good indication of the resolution of the abscess. When the discharge has reduced, the drains may be shortened or removed.

(i)   Maintain a six hourly temperature, pulse and respiration (TPR) chart.

(j)   Keep in hospital until the patient is apyrexic, the drains are out, and the drainage minimal.

5.   Make arrangements to eradicate the cause of the infection.

II INFLAMMATORY SWELLINGS SECONDARY TO PRIMARY PATHOLOGY

The inflammation may take three forms:

(a) Intra-oral ulceration which is secondarily infected. This occurs particularly where a malignancy erodes through the mucosa and allows oral organisms to proliferate in the necrotic tissue of the tumour.

(b) Direct spread of a primary tumour to cause a painful, inflammatory swelling which is red and painful to palpation, just beneath the skin surface. If left for a matter of days, the tumour will ulcerate through. Those who have not experienced this before may be tempted to incise and drain, with disastrous consequences of rapid fungation of tumour.

(c) Malignant spread to local lymph nodes which then become secondarily infected from ulceration in the primary tumour. These may present in the cervical nodes as tender, red and possibly suppurating swellings in the catchment area of the tumour.

Management

1. Identify the primary site by careful examination.
2. Take radiographs of any bony site which might be involved.
3. Determine the extent of the malignant process by CT scan and other appropriate tests, such as ultrasound, naso-endoscopy and examination under anaesthesia (EUA).

Remember that patients presenting with a first primary lesion in the mouth, may have a second primary lesion in the mouth and naso-pharynx. Look for it!

4. Take chest radiographs to ensure that the chest is clear of disease before embarking upon definitive treatment.
5. Determine the base-line state of the patient's blood — full blood picture, urea, electrolytes, and liver function tests as appropriate.
6. Take a fine needle aspiration biopsy or full histological biopsy under local analgesia, so as to be able to make a treatment plan as soon as possible.

III   NON-INFLAMMATORY SWELLINGS

Those that present acutely are few in number.

Angio-oedema

This may cause acute generalized swelling of the face. It is thought to be the result of allergy or as a response to insect bites and stings and is usually self-limiting. It is rare for oedema to spread and become life threatening but, *if there is a short history and a rapid increase in oedema, or if you are uncertain, admit to hospital for observation.*

Management

1.   Arrange for half-hourly observations by the nursing staff initially. The simplest way to do this is to ask for a half hourly TPR chart to be kept.
2.   Prescribe:

   (i)   Antihistamines. Chlopheniramine maleate, 4–8 mg orally or intramuscularly according to urgency. Repeat four to six hourly until the oedema is controlled.
   (ii)   Dexamethasone 8–16 mg intramuscularly. If the patient is in a state of shock, give the same dose intravenously. Repeat two, four, or six hourly according to response.

3.   Have a cricothyroidotomy and/or a tracheostomy set ready.
4.   Investigate the possible cause when the emergency is over.

Sialolithiasis

The most common salivary duct to become blocked by a stone is the submandibular, although the parotid is not exempt. The affected gland will enlarge at the thought, smell or sight of food. Such interference with normal salivary flow will encourage ascending infection. The patient may present with an enlarged painful gland with or without infection.

If the stone is evident by palpation and radiography, remove it under local anaesthesia, *but only if you have experience of the procedure.*

If you have not the experience, and you think that infection is complicating the swelling, prescribe antibiotics as above. Arrange for a sialogram. Ascending infection may progress to abscess formation. If this has occurred, proceed as above (page 128).

17: Emergency Management of Trauma in Hospital

GENERAL CONSIDERATIONS

As the patient arrives in the accident and emergency department, there are three major considerations — *airway, cervical spine,* and *blood loss.*

Although airway must be the first consideration, always consider that most injuries which cause damage to the facial skeleton involve flexion-extension manipulations to the cervical spine. These may cause a fracture and the cervical spine is potentially unstable. Manipulations to the neck therefore to improve the airway, must be done with this in mind.

Nursing the patient

The patient may be unconscious and, until facilities and equipment permit, should be nursed as near prone as possible. The patient is placed initially on his or her side, the uppermost leg is flexed at the hip and knee, the arm is flexed at the shoulder and elbow and the head is arranged with slight neck extension, and the mouth and nose as low as possible. The lower arm is extended posteriorly (*see* Fig. 17.1).

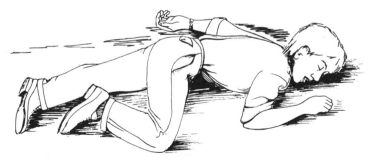

Fig. 17.1 The lower arm is extended posteriorly

Airway. If the patient remains *unconscious*, the position described above must be maintained until a good light and an aspirator are available. Before turning the patient on to the back however, a superficial examination should be made and the mouth thoroughly cleaned with an aspirator to remove blood clots, saliva and foreign bodies.

If the patient is *fully conscious*, and able to maintain his own airway he may be allowed to find his own comfortable position.

Where the patient is conscious and the blood pressure is being maintained, but *there is cause for concern* that the airway is at risk, nurse the patient in a semi-sitting position (Fig. 17.2). Here the trunk is kept at 45° to the horizontal with the head resting hard back on pillows. If the airway becomes embarrassed, the patient may simply lift the head forward a few degrees to protrude the tongue or clear the mouth of saliva or debris. This position reduces facial oedema, and may assist in preventing bleeding in the face or mouth by reducing the blood pressure in the head. Cot sides should be used on bed or trolley.

Even the severely injured may be nursed in this position. It should *not* be used where there is a possibility of a fracture cervical spine, or where the blood pressure is not being maintained.

Factors adversely affecting the airway

1. Unconsciousness.
2. Nursing the patient in the incorrect position.
3. Foreign bodies, blood clot, body fluids in the mouth and oropharynx, oedema or haematoma in the tongue and soft palate. The severely injured may have a haematoma along the posterior wall of the pharynx, and this may be suggestive of a fractured cervical spine.

Bear in mind: Oedema is progressive over hours. A patient presenting initially with a good airway may, within minutes, have the airway occluded by oedema or haematoma in the soft palate. This is uncommon but occurs particularly when there is:

4. Posterior impaction of the maxilla. A blow to the maxilla may separate the facial bones from the base of the skull, forcing them downwards and backwards. There is a false impression of a good oral airway due to an anterior open bite where the mandibular molars occlude prematurely on the upper molars which have been displaced downwards and backwards. All maxillary fractures cause occlusion of the nasal airway. A swollen soft palate may

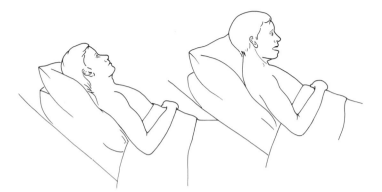

Fig. 17.2   The patient is nursed in a semi-sitting position

shut off the oral airway by contacting the posterior oropharyngeal wall and the posterior third of the tongue. This is particularly likely to occur where there are fractures of the mandible leading to swelling and haematoma in the tongue (Fig. 17.3).

Bear in mind: fractures of the mandible *never* cause occlusion of the airway simply by displacement of the insertions of the muscles of the tongue. If the airway becomes embarrassed, *improve the position of the patient.*

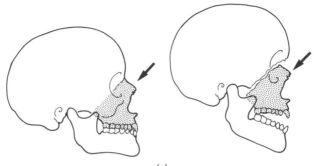

(a)

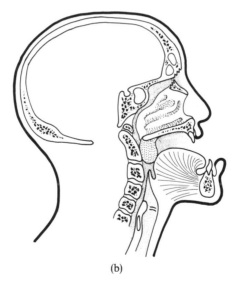

(b)

Fig. 17.3   (a) When a Le Fort III fracture is displaced by a blow from the front; it moves posteriorly and inferiorly. The impression is of a good oral airway as the patient has an anterior open bite. (b) Progressive oedema of the soft palate may occlude the airway by blocking of the nasal and oral airway.

I   THE UNCONSCIOUS PATIENT

1. Nurse the patient on the side (described above) until facilities are available for careful inspection.
2. Examine the mouth and oropharynx as far as possible with the patient in this position and aspirate the mouth and oropharynx, then
3. Roll the patient onto the back while still aspirating the mouth and oropharynx. As this is done maintain the patient's head and body in alignment in case there might be a fracture causing instability of the cervical spine. An assistant is usually required.
4. Under a good light, make a careful assessment as to the possible fractures, and the extent of oedema and haematomas. *Beware of the posteriorly displaced maxilla* (see above).
5. Insert a Brook Airway (or similar).
6. If the airway is adequate but it appears that it may deteriorate, consider intubating the patient immediately. Normally this is best left to the anaesthetic resuscitation team.
7. If the patient is deteriorating rapidly and skilled assistance is not available do a:
8. *Cricothyroidotomy.* Extent the neck, identify the lower border of the thyroid cartilage and the upper border of the cricoid cartilage immediately beneath, and insert five or six wide bore needles through the crycothyroid membrane. Most accident and emergency departments will have a special crycothyroid needle which is custom made for the purpose.

   This airway is generally adequate to gain time for more definitive procedures, such as a tracheostomy, to be done later.

II THE CONSCIOUS PATIENT

Where injuries permit, nurse in a semi-sitting position, with the trunk approximately 45° to the horizontal and the head held up on pillows (*see* Fig. 17.2).

Examination may be carried out in this position, as described above for the unconscious patient.

Cervical spine

Injuries to the facial skeleton almost always involve flexion-extension manipulations to the neck — the whiplash effect. Therefore, all patients with damage to the head and facial skeleton should be considered as having a fracture of the cervical spine. Where the patient is conscious, he or she will be able to protect a damaged cervical spine, whereas the unconscious patient will not. Special care therefore needs to be taken of the neck in all unconscious patients who have suffered recent trauma.

Whenever the patient is moved, the head and trunk must be moved simultaneously and the head and neck kept in the same plane. Therefore, two or more people must be available to move an unconscious patient. One person must be given prime responsibility for supporting the head and neck.

The conscious patient will experience pain in the neck such that the head will be held in the least painful position. On no account disturb this position by sudden movements during transport or examination, until you are satisfied that there is no cervical fracture present.

To examine the neck, assist the patient into a sitting position while supporting the neck. If there is restricted movement in any of these positions, arrange for cervical spine radiographs. *These should take precedence over all other radiographs except where life is threatened by damage to another system.*

Where a cervical spine fracture is suspected, immediately apply neck support with a foam collar.

Blood loss

Blood loss from the facial tissues may be dramatic, and occasionally may be life threatening. Many facial wounds are associated with damage to other parts of the body and haemorrhage into the tissues resulting from these may be hidden. Therefore, even though the injuries may appear to be restricted to the face, *examine the whole body*. This can be achieved satisfactorily only if all the patient's own clothes are removed. A scheme for assessing blood loss is shown in Figure 17.4. If it is considered that two units or more may have been lost proceed as follows:

1. Set up an intravenous line. In the process take blood for

    (a) Haemoglobin concentration
    (b) Blood group. If it is estimated that there is relatively minor blood loss ask for 'group and save'. This means that the blood will be grouped and the serum saved for a later crossmatch if necessary.
    (c) Crossmatch. If it is estimated that the blood loss is more than two units and may be progressive, request the preparation of two units of crossmatched blood. (Never ask for one unit; if you feel that one unit would be 'sufficient' it is unlikely that the patient requires transfusion).

2. Keep the line open with normal saline or Hartman's solution.
3. *Check antitetanus prophylaxis.*

For further information on management of blood loss *see* Chapter 18, page 153.

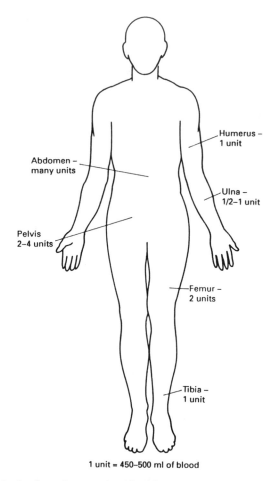

Humerus –
1 unit

Abdomen –
many units

Ulna –
1/2–1 unit

Pelvis
2–4 units

Femur –
2 units

Tibia –
1 unit

1 unit = 450–500 ml of blood

Fig. 17.4 A scheme for assessing blood loss.

III HEAD INJURY

Once the airway has been established, the cervical spine examined and assessed, the blood loss estimated and an intravenous drip set up if required, consideration must be given to the potential for head injury. *All trauma to the head or face, however slight, has potential for intracranial damage.*

History

1. If conscious, the patient should be asked details of the incident; where it occurred, how it occurred, from which direction the blow came, where did it strike?
2. What were the consequences of the injury? Was there a secondary blow to the head, did the patient fall down, how did the patient fall down?
3. If the patient has been unconscious, what was the last thing he remembers, what was he doing at the time? (Assessment of retrograde amnesia.)
4. Previous blows to the head. Past history may be important as previous injuries may leave residual signs which can confuse the examination in the new acute head injury.

If the patient is unconscious, take a history of the injury from bystanders and/or the ambulancemen who brought the patient to hospital. Has there been a lucid interval; has the patient's condition improved, declined or remained static?

Examination

(Eventually to include the whole body — which will require all clothes to be removed.)

1. Basic observations. *Record the time*, temperature, pulse, respiration, blood pressure — repeat these at 15 minute intervals if the patient is unconscious.
2. Examine for cerebrospinal fluid leak from the ears or nose.
3. Examine the whole cranium for lacerations and haematomata.
4. Examine for injury and stiffness of the neck. This should be done with extreme care until you are sure that there is no cervical spine fracture.
5. Examine for state of consciousness. Note the best motor response and verbal response the patient can manage. *Apply the coma scale*

in use in your hospital. If in doubt follow the Glasgow Coma scale (Table 17.2). Note the size of the pupils and their reaction to light.

Danger signs. (Parameters recorded at 15 minute intervals)

1. Consciousness — deepening level of coma
2. Ventilation — deepening breathing — slowing breathing — intervals of apnoea
3. Pupils — unilateral dilatation — decreased response to light — bilateral dilatation
4. Pulse — falling
5. Vomiting
6. Epileptic fits

Examine the whole body including the back and back of head for injury, lacerations, puncture wounds, etc.

Table 17.2   The Glasgow Coma scale

This gives a highly reliable way of recording the conscious state of a person. It can be used by medical, dental and nursing staff for initial and continuing assessment. It has a value also in predicting outcome. Three types of response are assessed:

Best motor response

This has five grades:

1. Carrying out request ('obeying command'): the patient does simple things you ask (beware of accepting the grasp reflex in this category).
2. Localizing response to pain: put pressure on the finger nail bed with a pencil. If the limb flexes, give a painful stimulus to the head, neck and trunk. A localizing response to pain is recorded if a painful stimulus at more than one site causes the patient to try to remove the stimulus by moving a limb.
3. Flexor response to pain: pressure on the nail bed causes flexion withdrawal of the limb.
4. Extensor posturing to pain: the stimulus causes limb extension (adduction, internal rotation of shoulder, pronation of the forearm).
5. No response to pain

NB. Record the best response of any limb.

Best verbal response

This has five grades:

1. Oriented: the patient knows who he is, where he is and why, the year, season and month.
2. Confused conversation: the patient responds to questions in a conversational manner but there is a degree of disorientation and confusion.
3. Inappropriate speech: random or exclamatory articulated speech, but no conversational exchange.
4. Incomprehensible speech: moaning but no words.
5. None.

NB. Record the best level of speech.

Eye opening.

This has four grades:

1. Spontaneous eye opening.
2. Eye opening in response to speech: any speech, or shout, not necessarily request to open the eyes.
3. Eye opening in response to pain: pain applied to limbs as above.
4. No eye opening.

IV   FACIAL INJURY

History

A history of the incident which caused the trauma is important. Particularly, try to find out what caused the blow and from which direction it came. Witnesses may be helpful.

Examination

(a) Shape of the face. Observe the face from different angles and assess for swelling, asymmetry and depression.

(b) Palpate the soft tissues gently to assess the extent of oedema, presence of surgical emphysema and foreign bodies.

(c) Palpate the facial skeleton; do this systematically.

- *Maxilla.* Supra-orbital ridges, bridge of nose, frontozygomatic suture, infra-orbital margin, zygomatic prominence, zygomatic arch, nasal septum.
- *Mandible.* Temporomandibular joints, posterior border of the mandible, inferior border of the mandible.
- *Intra-oral.* Occlusion of the teeth (the most valuable examination of all for maxillary and mandibular fractures). Run a gloved finger around the buccal sulcus in both jaws — the tuberosity, the zygomatic buttress, the piriform aperture; the external oblique ridge of the mandible, the labial sulcus. Examine with a good light for gingival lacerations and haematomata. In particular look for haematoma beneath the tongue.

(d) Examine for mobility (do not manipulate obvious fractures).

- *Maxilla.* Grasp the upper arch across the premolar area with one hand and the cranium across the frontal bone with the other, and attempt to detect movement vertically and horizontally between the two hands (rely on your own proprioception. Movements of the scalp over the cranium can give a false impression of bone mobility).
- *Mandible.* Grasp the mandible with each hand between the teeth and lower border, and attempt to 'spring' the mandible across suspected sites of fracture. Where there is suspicion of a fracture at the angle of the mandible, the ramus should be grasped in one hand and the body of the mandible in the other, and movement detected between the two hands by your own proprioception.

Bear in mind: This examination will require good light, if necessary held by an assistant, and an aspirator. Loose fragments of tooth or bone and foreign bodies may be removed during the intra-oral examination.

(e) Examine the eyes. If possible, part the lids to visualize the globes; note ecchymoses (always red under the conjunctiva), chemoses (conjunctival oedema), shape and position of the pupil, state of the iris.

- Sight — if conscious, ask the patient to count fingers or read large print; if unconscious, check pupil reactivity and cross-reactivity; if the lids are very swollen and cannot be prised apart, ask the conscious patient if a bright light can be detected in front of each eye.
- Movements — where possible, get the patient to follow the light of a pen torch, through the nine cardinal positions of gaze (straight forward, up, down, left, right, and the four oblique positions). Hold your torch not less than 1 metre away. Note any diplopia.

If in doubt about the condition of the globe of either eye, call the ophthalmologist on call.

Radiographs

1. *Maxilla*. To identify the fracture lines and to estimate displacement, the following will be required:
- Standard (10°) occipitomental taken postero-anterior (PA).
- Tilted (30°) occipitomental taken PA.
- Lateral of the facial bones, preferably with a 'wedge' across the nose to show possible fractures in the nasal bones.
- Submento-vertical, if there is doubt about a fractured zygomatic arch.

Bear in mind: — the ability to achieve these radiographs depends upon the general state of the patient, and is possible in many X-ray departments only if the patient is able to sit or stand. Some departments have a 'skull table' which enables PA radiographs to be taken with the patient lying on the back. Generally however, you will have to be content with AP radiographs until the patient is able to be turned or can sit. If fracture lines can be seen sufficient to make the diagnosis, do not insist on repeated views in the AP direction, as they will add little more information. Wait until the patient is fit enough to plan treatment, and arrange for the best views possible to be taken at that time, preferably PA. Ultimately tomograms or a CT scan may be required.

- Intra-oral radiographs — periapical and upper oblique occlusals are important where fractures of the alveolus and teeth are suspected.

2. *Mandible.* If the patient is able to sit or stand, arrange for the following radiographs:

  - Panoramic (orthopantomogram). This is ideal and is particularly good for showing up fractures of the mandibular condyle. At least one further view at right angles to a suspected fracture must be taken.
  - Postero-anterior (PA) of the facial bones — this will show fractures and lateral displacement in the ramus and sometimes of the condyle and condylar neck. Interpretation of fractures in the anterior region of the mandible is difficult.
  - Lateral of the facial bones — may help to clarify fractures in the anterior region of the mandible.
  - Reverse Townes — helps to define fractures of the condylar neck.
  - Intra-oral views — lower occlusal radiographs are valuable for fractures in the anterior region. Periapicals will reveal fractures of the alveolus and teeth.
  - Lateral oblique views are necessary where the patient is unable to stand or sit. Varying the angle of the beam will enable the whole mandible from condyle to the canine area to be seen. Interpretation of the fractures may be difficult and may require more than one view of each suspected fracture.

Bear in mind: the panoramic radiograph may be unsatisfactory for oblique fractures. Occasionally it is necessary to request tomograms.

3. *Chest.* It is *essential* to take radiographs of the chest where there is a possibility of a foreign body being inhaled; this is particularly important where teeth have been fractured and all the pieces have not been accounted for.

4. *Cervical spine.* Where a fracture of the cervical spine is suspected, arrange for:

  - Lateral
  - Postero-anterior
  - Postero-anterior of C2 with the mouth open (open mouth PA) to show the odontoid peg.

V   FRACTURED JAWS

Definitive treatment of fractured jaws requires good radiographs, with two views of each fracture, taken mutually at right angles. Not only do they identify the fracture, but the degree of displacement may be assessed. Frequently such radiographs may be taken only after the patient has been treated for the major injuries suffered. (*see* page 145).

All major injuries to a patient take precedence over the maxillofacial injuries, until:

(a)   The patient is stable, and the injuries have been assessed and most of them treated.

(b)   If certain that further anaesthetics will not be required — the airway must be clear for the anaesthetist.

Definitive treatment to the fractured facial bones should be left until the fractures may be fully assessed radiographically, and oedema of the face is subsiding. Sometimes it is helpful to prescribe Dexamethasone 8 mg twice a day to speed this process. Reduction of the fractures, particularly where bone plating or wiring becomes necessary, is far easier and a better result obtained. It is particularly important to delay surgery where possible, until the patient's condition is stable, when there will be a better chance of survival and a better likelihood of the patient achieving a normal life in the future. There is little point in achieving a beautiful cosmetic result on a patient who ends up decorticate, in renal failure, or in a coffin!

Description of the definitive treatment of fracture jaws is beyond the remit of this book. There are however, a number of things that must be done in the acute phase:

1.   All facial lacerations should be explored and sutured under local analgesia, where possible within hours of the injury, but certainly within 24 hours. The longer lacerations remain unsutured, the worse the scarring will be, and the greater the risks of secondary infection. Initially, the lacerations may be held together with steristips. If the patient is to be taken to the operating theatre for other reasons, the lacerations should be dealt with at the same time:

(a)   Debride and clean the wound. Explore and remove all foreign bodies.

(b)   Remove necrotic tissue, especially at the wound edges. Conserve all vital tissue.

(c) Restore tissue to its normal anatomical position. Minor
     tissue loss may be made up by undermining the skin or
     mucosa locally. Leave doubtful areas to those with expert-
     ise in the treatment of tissue loss; call them in if available.
(d) Suture. Approximate muscle with 3/0 chromic gut, the
     subcuticular tissues with 3/0 plain gut, the skin with 5/0
     monofilament material, and the mucosa with the same
     monofilament or 3/0 silk or 3/0 plain gut.

2. If the patient is to go to theatre by reason of other injuries, take
the opportunity to examine the patient under the anaesthetic and
reduce and hold the fractures in reasonable position. Occasionally,
it may be possible to use bone plates to complete the treatment
of, for instance a fractured mandible, but generally the minimum
should be done to make the patient comfortable in the least
possible time. If it is reasonable to hold the fracture by wiring
the teeth across the fracture line, do not rely on teeth adjacent
to the fracture line, use as many teeth as possible. Occasionally,
definitive treatment can be carried out.

*Under no circumstances, apply intermaxillary fixation unless you are
certain that the patient will have a good airway, that no further
anaesthetics will be required for at least three weeks, and that the
patient will go to the Intensive Care ward or have a special nurse over
the ensuing 12–24 hours.*

3. Give analgesics. Remember that the fractured maxilla is relatively
pain free, even when manipulated, whereas the mandible may be
excruciating!

(a) Aspirin is better avoided as it may encourage bleeding
     due to reduction of platelet aggregation. Paracetamol
     600–900 mg four hourly is often sufficient. Ibuprofen is
     an alternative, 400–600 mg six hourly.
(b) Pethidine 50–100 mg im according to weight, may be
     necessary for the fractured mandible. *Remember* that it
     may cause vomiting, it will cause constricted pupils and
     may mask signs of rising intracranial pressure, and it is a
     respiratory depressant. It is metabolized slowly where
     there is renal impairment.

*Never sedate the patient and, in particular, never prescribe papavaretum,
as it may be fatal.* There are occasions where sedation is advised, but
leave that to those in overall care of the patient.

Epistaxis

Trauma which fractures the middle third of the face or nasal bones will cause bleeding from the nose. Usually this is self-limiting, but occasionally becomes very worrying and will require treatment by a person experienced in its management. While waiting for such a person to arrive, a useful start may be made:

Treatment

1. Aspirate blood from the nose.
2. If the patient is conscious, spray the nasal mucosa with lignocaine and wait for two minutes. Examine with a nasal speculum and a good light. An auroscope is a good alternative.
3. If the bleeding seems to be close to the anterior nares, take a standard surgical glove, and cut around the base of the index and middle fingers, so that a 'pantaloon' is formed. Lubricate with KY jelly or liquid paraffin, and insert the 'fingers' up each nostril. Moisten a metre length of half inch (1 cm) ribbon gauze, and pack each end into the fingers so as to apply pressure to the nasal mucosa. Hold the packs in place with sticky tape around the base of the nose.
4. If the bleeding is severe, and arising more posteriorly from torn vessels in the fracture lines, conventional packing is impossible. Call for the assistance of an anaesthetist to provide sedation or even a general anaesthetic, and then pass a Foley catheter (available in all accident and emergency departments) down the nose so that the bulb lies in the nasopharynx. Blow up the bulb with approximately 10 ml of water, and pull the catheter forwards so that the bulb impacts in the posterior nares. A pack may be inserted in the nose against the bulb. Use half inch ribbon gauze soaked in Whitehead's varnish, or BIPP. Secure the catheter and pack. There are specially designed catheters available with two bulbs, one to impact against the posterior nares as above, the other to apply pressure within the nasal cavity.

    If the emergency is extreme, the above may have to be carried out with the patient unsedated.

18: Emergency Hospital Management of Haemorrhage

It is seldom that patients are referred to hospital having had all the measures outlined in Chapter 4 carried out. Thus, the hospital practitioner should begin by following the suggestions set out there to control the patient's bleeding by local measures. Prescribe antifibrinolytic agents, such as tranexamic acid, 1 g orally or by slow intravenous infusion. If these measures fail to control the bleeding within 30 minutes, further management will be necessary.

History

It is vital to take a full history which will include direct questions about the possible causes of an increased bleeding time (Table 18.1).

It is always wise to spend a few moments to discuss with relations, accompanying persons or ambulance men, the state of the patient over the past hour or so, so that an estimate can be made as to the total blood loss.

Bear in mind: a little blood goes a very long way, especially when diluted with saliva!

Take a blood sample. Where the bleeding is sufficiently severe to consider that there might be a systemic cause, take a blood sample by venepuncture sufficient for the following tests (approximately 10 ml):

(a) *Full blood picture* — this will include:

- Haemoglobin concentration
- Mean corpuscular haemoglobin concentration
- White cell count
- Platelet count

State the reasons for the test clearly on the request form, so that the laboratory will recognize which tests need to be done first amongst the many that are usually carried out. This is particularly so at night, where automated systems may not be running. This investigation gives a baseline reading of the haemoglobin, but it must be remembered that this may overstate the value if bleeding has been brisk, because

Table 18.1   Some causes of increased bleeding time

1. *Clotting defects*

- (a)   Haemophilia A (reduced factor VIII)
- (b)   Von Willebrand's disease (reduced factor VIII and reduced platelet adhesion factor)
- (c)   Haemophilia B (reduced factor IX, Christmas disease)
- (d)   Anticoagulants (heparin, warfirin)
- (e)   Liver disease

2.   *Platelet aggregation defects*

- (a)   Thrombocytopenia
  Reduced production

  - Leukaemia
  - Myelofibrosis
  - Drugs
  - Toxins
  - Irradiation
  - Viral illnesses (glandular fever)

- (b)   Reduced survival

  - Idiopathic thrombocytopenic purpura
  - Drug induced
  - Disseminated intravascular clotting (associated with other factors in severe trauma).

- (c)   Reduced platelet function

  - Acute alcohol intoxication
  - High aspirin intake
  - Excessive transfusion with dextrans

3.   *Vessel wall defects*

- (a)   Hereditary haemorrhagic telangiectasia
- (b)   Ehlers–Danlos syndrome
- (c)   Henoch-Schonlein purpura
- (d)   Cushing's disease
- (e)   Long-term steroid therapy
- (f)   Aging skin and mucosa

4.   *Local effects*

Local inflammation as in chronic gingivitis. This has vessel wall effects superimposed upon vasodilatation, and increased fibrinolysis.

haemodilution has not taken place fully. In general terms, each reduction of one g/100 ml in Hb below the normal (14.8 g for males, 13.8 g for females) represents 500–600 ml of blood lost.

Platelet count — it is essential to know the numbers of platelets per ml of blood where thrombocytopaenia is suspected. Unsuspected thrombocytopaenia is not uncommon however, and hence the request is mandatory.

(b) *'Group and save'*. *It is essential* that blood is taken early for blood grouping, with sufficient to do a cross-match, if necessary. Should the patient's condition deteriorate, it becomes increasingly difficult to enter a vein for a venepuncture, as the patient becomes more nervous and may even become shocked.

The veins collapse, and the arm becomes as unrewarding as a stone.

The second reason, and equally important, is that colloid substitutes for blood which may be used to restore blood volume, make it difficult or impossible to group and cross-match blood at a later stage.

(c) *Screen for a bleeding diathesis*. Until recently, each haematology department has had its own standard tests for bleeding tendency. If in doubt request 'screen for bleeding tendency'. The result will be given as INR (International Normalizing Ratio). Each laboratory however, interprets the results a little differently. Generally, the tested blood is set against a standard, and 'normal' is taken in the range 1:1 to 1.5:1. Any value above this is abnormal, with a bleeding tooth socket difficult to control at 3:1, and spontaneous uncontrolled bleeding occurring at 5:1.

Intravenous infusion. While taking blood for the above investigations and if the patient has lost a lot of blood already, it may be worthwhile setting up an intravenous 'drip' at the same time. Consider it. Keep open with a slow infusion of normal saline (10 drips per minute) until the patient's condition improves.

Sedate the patient. One of the most potent causes of bleeding is anxiety. Anxiety raises the blood pressure and increases fibrinolytic activity. Patient agitation will disturb clot formation. Reassurance will help. Strict and severe instructions may be required to prevent the patient interfering with the formation of the clot. If it is felt that the patient is likely to remain as an outpatient and is to go home within an hour or so, mild sedation with diazepam (10 mg) or temazepam (20–30 mg) orally may be sufficient. If in doubt:

Admit to hospital. A short stay ward, or 24-hour ward, is ideal if there is one available to you.

Now, sedation may be increased. Papaveretum (Omnopon), 10–20 mg intramuscularly according to weight and agitation, usually suffices. Pethidine 75–100 mg intramuscularly is an alternative.

When the patient is calm, examine the mouth once more, and carry out any necessary local measures while awaiting the return of any blood tests which have been requested. If there appears to be an arterial bleed, transfer the patient to a minor operating suite or surgery, where there is a good light, good aspiration and competent assistance. *Do not* attempt to treat the patient on a bed in an ill-lit ward. As appropriate, insert more local anaesthetic containing adrenaline, identify the bleeding point, raise a flap if necessary, and apply diathermy. Bipolar diathermy is best and safest. If unipolar diathermy only is available, take stringent precautions not to burn the patient. Re-suture and re-apply local measures as outlined in Chapter 4. In rare instances, it may be necessary to arrange for a general anaesthetic.

If a bleeding diathesis is identified, call for the assistance of a haematologist or appropriate medical firm to manage the clotting problem. Do not be tempted to dabble in medical management, apart from prescribing fibrinolytic agents, as set out above. *Never* be persuaded to tie off feeding arteries to an area where bleeding is occurring, until the INR is approaching the normal range, because surgical intervention will only promote further bleeding.

19:   Emergencies Involving the Oral Mucous Membranes — Hospital Management

Details of the conditions which can affect the oral mucous membranes will be found in Chapter 5. Preliminary treatment is described, but ultimately, most will be referred to a hospital department of oral surgery/oral medicine. Here, it is *essential* to establish a diagnosis before progressing to more complex treatments. Where there is any doubt about the possible diagnosis:

Take a biopsy

Inject local anaesthetic solution beneath the lesion, avoiding the area to be biopsied. This ensures that there is no damage to the biopsy itself. After the area is anaesthetized, take a specimen which contains normal and abnormal tissue, and the interface between the two. A common mistake is to make the section too shallow. Usually, the specimen is in the form of an ellipse. Place the tissue immediately in formol saline, and ensure that the specimen bottle is marked with the patient's name and hospital number, and is dated. Fill in a request form, similarly marked.

Where immune studies are to be performed, a second biopsy should be taken next to the first. It might seem that it is easier to take one larger biopsy and bisect it to produce two specimens. In practice, orientation of the specimen is lost as it is cut in half, so that oblique slices result. Subsequent interpretation of these sections is difficult. The second biopsy is immersed immediately in liquid nitrogen, usually by a pathology technician. Where the tissue is very friable, and the surface epithelium readily strips off, a biopsy from apparently unaffected mucosa may give better information. Never hesitate to take tissue from more than one place if necessary. A blood sample may be required for indirect immunofluorescence, where pemphigus and mucous membrane pemphigoid are suspected.

Some laboratories are satisfied with a punch biopsy, but a generous incisional biopsy is generally considered more satisfactory.

Blood tests

Many oral mucosal lesions may be associated with abnormal results in blood tests.

1. *Full blood picture (FBP)* — this includes:

- Haemoglobin concentration
- Mean corpuscular volume
- Mean corpuscular haemoglobin concentration (MCHC)
- White cell count and differential
- Platelet count

This gives an overall picture of the state of the cellular component of the patient's blood. Where readings vary from the normal, some laboratories will report on a blood smear to detect abnormalities in the shape and size of the cells — macrocytes, where the MCHC is low in the presence of anaemia, for instance. It may have to be requested separately.

2. *Erythrocyte Sedimentation Rate (ESR)*. This is still a valuable test. Being non-specific, it is an indicator that 'something may be wrong'.
3. *Serum iron and iron binding capacity*. Serum iron may be low and the binding capacity high in many diseases of the oral mucous membranes; for example candidiasis, ulcerations, bullous lesions, sore mouth from any cause.
4. *Serum B_{12}*. Sore mouth and tongue may be signs of B_{12} deficiency. Patients who are over 40 and who are approaching the age where pernicious anaemia is seen should be tested for possible B_{12} deficiency before asking for serum iron levels. This avoids unnecessary expenditure. It must be remembered that overt pernicious anaemia does not develop until late middle age, and that changes in the oral mucous membranes may be the first sign. Where the serum B_{12} level is low, the test should be followed up with a test for gastric parietal cell antibodies, which will differentiate between a dietary deficiency and the full syndrome of pernicious anaemia including achlorhydria and the risk of gastric carcinoma. The patient should be referred to a physician.
5. *Serum folate*. This is an imprecise test but may be a useful indicator of a dietary deficiency or malabsorption. A high level may represent a high level intake at a recent meal, but then this makes deficiency unlikely. Where there is reason to suspect that the oral condition may be associated with malabsorption, red-

cell folate may be requested. This is an expensive test but gives a more accurate estimate of the body stores. If low, malabsorption may be suspected.

Bear in mind: Where there is a low red cell folate and a low serum B_{12}, *never* give folate until after the first injection of B_{12}, and the commencement of a course of iron, for the patient's condition of pernicious anaemia may be pushed rapidly into the full syndrome with rapid degeneration in the neurological signs, which may be irreversible.

6. *Specific tests.*

   (a) Bullous lesions. Direct and indirect immunofluorescence, to detect antibodies against oral skin and mucous membranes.
   (b) Lupus erythematosus. Lichen planus and discoid or systemic lupus erythematosus may look very similar. Where there is suspicion that lupus erythematosus could be the cause, test for the presence of antinuclear factor.
   (c) Tests to exclude systemic causes — for example, fasting blood sugar (and urinalysis) for diabetes.

Treatment

Local treatment has been discussed in Chapter 5 for the individual conditions. Hospital treatment will follow along the same lines.
Systemic treatment. Generalized systemic disease, causing local oral manifestations, will require the involvement of other specialities to treat the acute condition. For example, oral candidiasis associated with poorly controlled diabetes, can only be treated in association with the appropriate medical firm, and oral purpura associated with thrombocytopenia in association with the department of haematology. Thus, generalized disease causing the acute oral condition must be excluded before further hospital treatment is contemplated by the department of oral medicine/surgery alone.

   (a) *Hospital admission.* Herpes zoster and erythema multiforme may require hospital admission. The oral lesions may be so painful that the patient becomes dehydrated from poor fluid intake and high fluid loss (where there is a significant pyrexia). Patients suffering acute herpes zoster should be admitted to an isolation ward, those with erythema multiforme need not. An intravenous infusion should be set up, with a fluid regime providing 3 L/day of 50:50 normal saline/Hartman's solution.

Other acute conditions of the oral mucous membranes may have systemic effects which require management in co-operation with medical specialist firms. Pemphigus is an example.

(b) *Analgesics.* The patient may be made comfortable by peripherally acting analgesics such as aspirin and paracetamol. If the pain is not controlled sufficiently, aspirin and papaveretum compound effervescent tablets taken four hourly, are a little stronger. Narcotic analgesics are seldom required.

(c) *Steroids.* Before systemic steroids are administered, it is *essential* that a history of peptic ulceration and diabetes are excluded; it is unwise to prescribe steroids where there is a history of tuberculosis, or where there is any sign of overt infection. Thus, systemic steroids should be restricted to ulcerative and bullous lesions, uncomplicated by any other medical conditions. Their effect to produce a rapid relief of symptoms may be dramatic.

Oral prednisolone is the drug of choice. A short course starting at 60 mg per day in divided doses, and reducing to nil in eight days, is sufficient for most ulcerations (see schedule in Table 19.1)

Table 19.1   A scheme for a short reducing course of oral steroid

Prednisolone 5 mg tablets

Day	Time				Dosage
	0700	1300	1700	2200	
Day 1	3	3	3	3	(60 mg)
Day 2	3	3	3	3	(60 mg)
Day 3	3	3	3	3	(60 mg)
Day 4	2	2	2	2	(40 mg)
Day 5	2	1	2	1	(30 mg)
Day 6	1	1	1	1	(20 mg)
Day 7	1	0	1	0	(10 mg)
Day 8	0	0	0	0	(0 mg)

20: Sedation Emergencies in Practice and Hospital

Sedation of patients prior to dental and oral surgical procedures is becoming increasingly popular. Not only are patients less anxious and more cooperative, but they have amnesia for the event and are thus more prepared to have further treatment by this means in the future. However, before considering treating a patient using sedation, a good understanding of the sedation agent is essential, and the surgery must be equipped with resuscitatory apparatus as described in Chapter 6. Flumazenil, a specific benzodiazepine antagonist, must be available when benzodiazepines are being used.

The current guidelines for dental practitioners issued by the General Dental Council (General Dental Practice 1988) demand, as a minimum requirement, that a second suitably-trained person is present throughout the procedure, who is capable of monitoring the clinical condition of the patient. This may be a dental surgery assistant or auxillary who must be present until the patient's protective reflexes have returned and be capable of assisting the dentist in case of emergency. The dental practitioner must be suitably experienced and take full responsibility for sedating the patient using a drug or drugs which produce a state of depression of the central nervous system, but during which communication is maintained such that the patient will respond to command. The drugs and techniques used should carry a margin of safety wide enough to render the unintended loss of consciousness unlikely. The following recommendations apply equally to hospital practice.

In view of these guidelines, sedation in dental practice at the present time should be restricted to the use of the benzodiazepines or relative analgesia. Relative analgesia will be considered later.

Bear in mind: Even though sedated, the patient may still faint. It is advisable always to treat the patient in the supine or near-supine position when sedation is used.

Sedating agents may give patients hallucinations. For the protection of the dentist and staff, two persons should be present at all times while the patient is sedated, so that events may be corroborated.

I BENZODIAZEPINES

It must be remembered that all benzodiazepines are respiratory depressants, and should be avoided in respiratory and cardiovascular disease. They should be avoided in alcohol abusers.

These may be given orally and intravenously. Rarely a combination of oral and intravenous routes may be used, but this is best avoided.

1. Oral sedation. This may be given as a small dose to render the patient less nervous, preparing them for dental or oral surgery, or in a relatively large dose to produce profound sedation for the actual procedure.

- Mild sedation — diazepam 5 mg the night before the procedure, 5 mg in the morning and, if necessary, 5 mg 1 hour before the procedure. The very nervous may require twice this amount, but it is advisable to check with the patient's medical practitioner before prescribing this dose. A small dose (less than half the usual) of intravenous agent may be used in addition in some circumstances just prior to the procedure, but should be administered slowly and with extreme care. The combination is best avoided.

- Profound sedation — temazepam 20–30 mg one hour before the dental or oral surgical procedure. *This must never be followed by intravenous sedation as the respiratory depressive effects are unpredictable.*

2. Intravenous sedation. The GDC guidelines should be followed. *Always use an intravenous canula or 'butterfly', as these give immediate access to a vein if complications should arise.* The agent should be given with the patient supine, slowly over 1–2 minutes and *never* as a bolus. The lid-lag sign (ptosis) is unpredictable. The best way to assess the effects of the sedating agent is to question the patient and note the replies. Slightly slurred and hesitant speech usually denotes sufficient drug.

The two main preparations in common use are diazepam and midazolam. Midazolam has a half-life of a little over 60 minutes, and the patient recovers more rapidly than with diazepam (half-life 21–40 hours), but there is a greater incidence of respiratory depression, and profound hypotension has been reported. There is little to choose between the recovery from the two drugs clinically however in the doses normally used for sedation, as both are rapidly protein-bound and removed from the circulation. Patients already taking oral preparations behave unpredictably.

- *Diazepam* 10–20 mg intravenously according to patient response.

The injections tend to be painful and there is a high incidence of venous thrombosis which occurs up to a week later. Consequently, it has been replaced by:

- *Diazemuls* 10–20 mg intravenously slowly according to patient response.
- *Midazolam* 2.5–7.5 mg by slow intravenous injection according to patient response. The preparation containing 2 mg per ml is advised as titration of the correct dose is easier than the more concentrated preparation of 5 mg per ml.

Never administer a benzodiazepine to a patient already receiving a drug known to be a respiratory depressant – such as pethidine or alcohol.

The dental surgeon and assistant must watch the patient at all times for signs of respiratory depression. These are:

1. Slow or intermittent breathing. Occasionally breathing may cease altogether (apnoea).
2. A pale or dusky skin. Cyanosis may be apparent.

The emergency

1. Lay the patient on their side.
2. Check that the patient has a clear and unobstructed airway. If necessary, insert a Brook airway (or similar).

    If it is apparent that the patient has a clear and unobstructed airway yet there is respiratory embarrasment and the cause is likely to be the benzo-diazepine, then:
3. Inject Flumazenil intravenously. This is a specific benzodiazepine antagonist. Inject 200 μg immediately over 15 s and, if the desired level of reversal is not achieved in 1 min, inject further doses of 100 μg at 60 s intervals to a maximum of 1 mg. The usual dose is 300–600 μg.
4. If rapid recovery occurs, *keep the patient under close observation.* Elimination of flumazenil is rapid and its half-life is less than 1 hour. If midazolam has been the sedating agent, a return of complications is unlikely. Diazepam has a far longer half-life than flumazenil and, if it is thought or known that the sedation was induced by this agent, further doses of flumazenil may be required as sedation and respiratory depression may recur. *It is essential that the patient should never be left alone without the dentist or assistant being present until the full dose of benzodiazepine taken over the previous 24 hours has been established beyond reasonable doubt.*

5. Closely question the patient and/or relative during the recovery phase as to whether unreported diazepam had been taken in the last 24 hours. If the answer is affirmative and the dose, in any form exceeds 30 mg., *or if there are doubts about long-term recovery*, call an ambulance and refer to the local accident and emergency department.

6. If you are confident that the patient has not had more than the dose of benzodiazepine known to you, and that this is not more than the recommended dose, the patient may be discharged home after 90 minutes. Where doubt exists, consult with the patient's general practitioner or refer to hospital by telephone.

II   RELATIVE ANALGESIA

Nitrous oxide has powerful analgesic properties and has been used in obstetric practice for many years. Currently it is dispensed as a 50:50 mixture with oxygen (Entonox) which produces analgesia without loss of consciousness. It is self-administered using a mask and demand valve and, if the patient becomes over-sedated, the mask falls from the face and recovery follows. As a large mask covering the mouth is inappropriate for use with dentistry, small nose masks are available, but these have to be fixed to the patient's face and the gas cannot be self-administered by the patient. Machines have become available to the dental profession whereby the proportion of nitrous oxide is variable, as decided by the dentist, but the concentration of oxygen is never less than 21%. The technique has become known as Relative Analgesia.

Recovery from sedation follows a few breaths of oxygen or air, as nitrous oxide is rapidly replaced in the lung and blood by oxygen. Hence it is a very safe technique, provided that the machine is performing optimally. *The machine should be serviced by a properly qualified person annually.*

Emergencies in relative analgesia

These are rare.

1. Excessive sedation – administer pure oxygen or remove the mask and allow the patient to breathe air. To continue the procedure, reduce the concentration of nitrous oxide.
2. Nausea and vomiting. Some patients seem prone to nausea and rarely, vomiting may follow. Remove the mask, or administer pure oxygen, and turn the patient on the side, taking precautions to avoid the patient's aspirating the vomit. Adjust the dental chair so that the head is lower than the thorax.

Loss of an instrument or foreign body during sedation

In all sedative techniques and in Relative Analgesia, the cough reflex should be maintained and thus the chances of aspiration of oral fluids, and of disappearance foreign bodies such as a piece of filling or instrument, are little more than that for the conscious patient. In this event however:

1. Maintain the sedation and thoroughly aspirate the mouth and oropharynx.
2. Adjust the dental chair so that the patient's head is lower than the thorax, and repeat the procedure.
3. Stop the sedation and turn the patient on the side, until recovery from the effects of the sedation is complete. Where a benzodiazepine has been used, reverse the sedation using fluma-zenil (see above).
4. Proceed as in Chapter 14.

REFERENCES

General Dental Council. (1988). Professional conduct and fitness to practise. *Notice for the guidance of dentists*, May.

Appendix

Commonly used Antibiotics available in the Dental Practitioners formulary

Phenoxymethyl Penicillin (Penicillin V) 250–500 mg four times per day orally. A useful and cheap drug where the patient is not sensitive to penicillin. Heavily protein-bound and suitable for mild to moderate infections only.

Benzyl Penicillin 600 mg four times per day by intramuscular injection. Ideal in severe infections where the patient is not penicillin sensitive, but its use is generally restricted to hospital. Use when the patient is unlikely to be able to absorb an oral antibiotic (assume this if the pyrexia is over 38.5°C).

Amoxycillin 250–500 mg three time per day, or 3G sachet daily orally. Ideal in the ambulant patient with a severe infection, where there is no penicillin sensitivity and only a moderate pyrexia. Can be used with Metronidazole in severe or potentially dangerous infections.

Cephradine 250–500 mg four times per day orally. Intramuscular injection available (500 mg vial). A useful second-line drug where there is a history of mild penicillin sensitivity. *Never prescribe where there is a history of severe penicillin sensitivity with anaphylactic reactions etc.* as there may be cross reactivity.

Cephalexin 250–500 mg four times per day orally. Similar to Cephradine but cannot be given by injection.

Clindamycin 150–300 mg four times per day orally, or as injection. This is a useful second-line antibiotic where mixed Gram-positive and – negative infection is suspected. If diarrhoea complicates the illness, *stop the drug immediately.* Clindamycin may cause pseudo-membranous colitis which can be fatal.

Co-trimoxazole A mixture of sulphamethoxazole and trimethoprim (5:1). 960 mg (2 tablets) twice per day orally. Useful in mild infections only.

Erythromycin 250–500 mg four times per day orally. A useful second-line drug in the penicillin-sensitive patient in mild infections. Absorbtion and protein-binding render it less effective than the penicillins, weight for weight.

Metronidazole 200–400 mg three times per day orally. Ideal in most infections in the oro-facial region, particularly where there is a history of penicillin sensitivity. Nausea is stimulated by alcohol, but some patients become unable to tolerate it even without alcohol. It may be given by suppository, 500–1000 mg every 8 hours. In severe infections, but where the patient is ambulant and with a pyrexia of less than 38.5°C, it is wise to add amoxycillin.

Oxytetracycline 250–500 mg four times per day orally. A useful alternative to the penicillins in mild to moderate infections. *Never* prescribe to children until the crowns of the teeth are complete.

Index

Acoustic neuroma 12
Acquired immune deficiency
    syndrome (AIDS), hairy
    leukoplakia in 51
Acrylic provisional crown
    problems 80
Acute herpetic gingivostomatitis
    96
Acute marginal gingivitis 95
Acute necrotising ulcerative
    gingivitis (Vincent's infection)
    95
Acute periapical abscess 16–17,
    88–9
Acute periodontal abscess
    17–18, 94–5
Acute swellings, management in
    hospital
    non-inflammatory swellings
        132–3
    primary inflammatory
        swellings 128–9
    secondary inflammatory
        swellings 131–2
Adrenocortical insufficiency
    (Addisonian crisis) 67–8
Airway, factors adversely
    affecting 134–5
Alveolar process fracture 110
Anaphylaxis 66–7
Angina 63
Angina haemorrhagica bullosa
    recurrens 48
Angio-oedema 23, 132–3
Angular cheilitis 52–3

Anterior tooth crown fracture
    33
Anterior tooth root fracture 33
Anticoagulants 35
Aphthous ulceration 42–3
Aspirin 35
    chemical burn 51
Asthma attack 69
Atypical facial pain 13, 125
Atypical odontalgia 14, 126

Behçet's syndrome 43
Benzodiazepines emergencies
    158–61
    intravenous sedation 159–60
    oral sedation 159
Berry aneurysm rupture 61
Bleeding time, causes of
    increase 151 (table)
Blood loss 138
    assessment 140
Blows 116
Boils 22
Broken needles 114–16
Broken rotatory instrument
    113–14
Broken shoulder joint 86
Bullous (blistering) lesions
    44–48

Candida albicans 52–4
Candidiasis, acute 52–3, 100
    diabetes associated 156
Cardiorespiratory arrest 57
    (table)
Carpopedal spasm 68

Cellulitis (Ludwig's angina) 24–5
Cerebrovascular accident (stroke) 61
Cervical spine injury 133–4, 138–9
Cervical sensitivity 79
Chest pain 63–65
Child abuse 72–5
  actions to be taken 74–5
  dentist's responsibility 72
  signs/recognition 72–4
Christmas disease 35–6
Cluster headache (periodic migrainous neuralgia) 10 123–4
Completely avulsed tooth 32–3
Cracked tooth 7–8, 89
Cranial arteritis 12, 124
Cricothyroidotomy 137
Crohn's disease 53
Crown dislodged by fracture of preparation 83–4

Degloving injury 28
Dental floss trauma 96
Dentine hypersensitivity 98
Diabetic coma:
  hyperglycaemic 60–1
  hypoglycaemic 60
Diazemuls 160
Diazepam 159–160
Discomfort on biting 77–8
Dissecting aneurysm 65
Drug–induced gingival hyperplasia 97

Emergency medication (table) 55
Emergency oxygen (table) 55
Endodontic emergencies 87
  before commencing treatment 87–9
  during treatment 90–91
    fractured instrument 90
    inadequate analgesia 90
    incomplete canal preparation 90–1
    perforation of root 90
  following treatment 92
    high restoration 92
    infected pulp tissue/debris in canal 92
    overfilling 92
    root fracture 92
    underfilling 92
  inhalation/swallowing of instrument 87
  primary dentition 93
Entonox 162
Epileptic fit 58–9
  avoidance 59
Epistaxis 149
Erythema migrans (geographic tongue) 51–2
Erythema multiforme 45
  treatment 156–7
External swellings, acute 21–3
  generalized swelling of facial tissues 24
  haematoma 22
  infectious fevers 22
  lymph nodes 21
  mucous extravasation cyst 22–3
  salivary glands 22
  skin 22
  tumours 22

Facial injury 144–5
  radiographs 145–6
Facial pain:
  atypical 13, 125
  bilateral dull 13, 125–7

clinical examination 3
diagnostic scheme (table) 2
emergency hospital treatment
     119–27
history 1–3
iatrogenic causes 8–9
special tests 3
tumours causing *see under*
     tumours
unilateral dull 5, 121–4
unilateral sharp 4–5, 119–20
Faint 56–8
Falls 116
Febrile convulsion 59
Flumazemil 158
Folate deficiency 15–16
Foreign body, small, in soft
     tissues 114–16
Fractured complete denture 102
Fractured endodontic
     instrument 90
Fractured jaw 109–10
     alveolar process 110
     mandible 111
         pathological 22
     treatment 147–9
Fractured porcelain 82–3
Fractured post 85
Fractured restoration 7

Galvanic restoration 79
Geographic tongue (erythema
     migrans) 51–2
Gingival abscess 18
Gingival discomfort 77
Gingival irritation proliferation
     under pontic 86
Gingival swellings, systemic
     disorders 97
Gingivitis:
     acute marginal 95
     acute necrotizing ulcerative
         43, 95–6
Gingivostomatitis, acute
     herpetic 96
Glandular fever 21, 22
Glasgow Coma Scale (table)
     143
Glossopharyngeal neuralgia 5,
     119
Granuloma:
     pyogenic 15
     traumatized denture 15

Haematoma 19
     extraoral 23
Haemophilia 35–6
Haemorrhage from mouth 35–9
     drugs causing 35
     emergency hospital
         management 150–3
         admission 153
         blood grouping 152
         blood tests 150–1
         history 150
         intravenous infusion 152
         screening for bleeding
             diathesis 152
         sedation 152
     post-extraction 36–9
Haemorrhagic telangiectasia,
     hereditary 49
Hairy leukoplakia 51
Head injury 141–4
Hepatitis B (HBV) patients 70–1
Herpes simplex 44
     secondary 44–5
Herpes zoster 11, 45–6
     admission to hospital 153
     treatment 122–3, 156–7
Herpetic gingivostomatitis 44,
     96
Hiatus hernia 64
High restoration 92

HIV infection 70–1
Hyperkeratosis 51
Hyperventilation 68

Iatrogenic trauma 109–19
  blows 116
  broken needle 114–16
  broken rotary instrument
    113–14
  falls 116
  fractured jaw *see* fractured
    jaw
  lacerations 109
  oro–antral fistula 111–13
  small foreign body in soft
    tissues 114–16
Immediate replacement denture
  102–3
  prosthodontic phase
    problems 103
  surgical phase problems 103
Inadequate approximal contact
  problems 78–9
Inferior alveolar block injection
  complications 116–17
International Normalizing
  Ratio 152
Intraoral swellings, acute 15–16

Kaposi's sarcoma 53

Lacerations 109
Leukaemia 36
Leukoplakia 51
Lichen planus 51, 156
Lips 52
  cracked 52–3
  swollen 53
Ludwig's angina (cellulitis) 24–5
Lupus erythematosus 156

Malabsorption syndrome 42–3

Malignant ulcer 41
Measles 21
Medical emergencies 55–69
Melkersson-Rosenthal
  syndrome 53
Midazolam 160
Mucous extravasation cyst 22
Mumps 22
Myocardial ischaemia/infarction
  63–4

Nikolsky sign 47
Nitrous oxide 162
Non-accidental injury *see* child
  abuse

Odontalgia, atypical 14, 126–7
Oral dysaesthesia complex 53
Oral mucous membrane lesions
  154–7
  biopsy 154
  blood tests 155–6
  treatment 156–7
Oro–antral fistula 15, 111–13
Orofacial tissue swellings 24–5
  alae of nose 25
  angle of mandible 24
  anterior mandible, chin 24
  body of mandible 24
  cheeks 25
  generalized swelling of neck
    24–5
  lower lip 25
  periorbital 25
  side of neck 24
  upper lip 25
Orthodontic emergencies 106–8
  external trauma 108
  fixed appliances 107–8
    fractured/displaced wires
      108
    loose attachments 107

loose bands 107
loose ligaments 108
pain 108
removable appliances 106
broken acrylic bases 106
broken wire components 106
distorted wire components 107
Orthopantomogram 146

Parotid gland enlargement 22
Paroxysmal trigeminal neuralgia 5, 119–20
Partial denture:
fracture of major connector 104
immediate addition 104
loss of function of clasp 104
Partially avulsed tooth 31
Pathological fracture of mandible 22
Pemphigoid 47
Pemphigus 46–7
Perforation of root 20, 90
Periapical abscess 6, 16–17
Pericarditis 65
Periocoronitis 18–19
Periodic migrainous neuralgia (cluster headache) 10, 123–4
Periodontal abscess, acute 17–18, 94–5
Periodontal emergencies 94–8
abscess formation 94–5
dentine hypersensitivity 98
postoperative bleeding 98
postoperative infection 97
Peritonsillar abscess (quinsy) 20
Phenytoin 97
Platelet disorders 36
Pneumothorax 65
Pontic, gingival irritation

proliferation under 86
Porcelain repair kit 82
Posterior tooth crown fracture 34
Posterior tooth root fracture 34
Post–extraction haemorrhage 36–9
Pregnancy epulis 15
Prosthodontic emergencies 99–105
fractured complete denture 102
immediate replacement denture see immediate replacement denture
new complete denture 99–102
cheek biting 101–2
generalized inflammation
localized bruising/ulceration on denture-bearing mucosa 100
localized bruising/ulceration related to periphery 100–1
palatal ulceration 101
partial denture fracture see partial denture
Provisional bridge problems 81
Pulmonary embolism 65
Pulpitis 5
irreversible 7, 8
reversible 4, 87–8
Purpura 49
thrombocytopenic 49
Pyogenic granuloma 15

Quinsy (peritonsillar abscess) 20

Ranula 15
Relative analgesia 158
emergencies 158, 162
Respiratory depression signs 159

Respiratory emergencies 68–9
Restorative emergencies 76–86
  problems following placement
    of restoration 76–7
    cervical sensitivity 79
    galvanic restoration 79
    gingival discomfort 77
    inadequate approximal
      contact 78–9
    thermal sensitivity 76–7
  problems of existing crowns/
    fixed bridgework 80–86
    acrylic provisional crown
      80
    broken shoulder joint 86
    crown dislodged by
      fracture of preparation
      83
    fractured porcelain 82–3
    fractured post 85
    gingival irritation
      proliferation under
      pontic 86
    provisional bridges 81
    uncemented bridge retainer
      85
    uncemented crown 83
    uncemented post crown
      84–5
Reticuloses 22
Red mouth 53
Root fracture following
  endodontic treatment 90
Root perforation 19–20

Salicylate overdose 68
Salivary gland enlargement 22
Sebaceous cyst 21
Sedation emergencies 158–61
  loss of instrument/foreign
    body in oral cavity 162
Self-inflicted gingival/mucosal

  injuries 96–97
Shingles see herpes zoster
Shock 66–7
Sialolithiasis 132
Sinusitis 125
Staphyloccocal infection of
  lymph nodes 21
Steroids 157
Stomatitis artefacta 40–1
Stroke (cerebrovascular
  accident) 61–2
Submandibular gland 22
Suppurative parotitis 22
Surgical emphysema 23–4
Suturing set 37 (fig.)

Teething 54
Temporomandibular (TM) joint
  dysfunction 10–11, 121–2
Thermal sensitivity 76–7
Thrombocytopenia 36
Thrombocytopenic purpura 48,
  151
Toothbrush trauma 96
Tracheitis 63
Transient ischaemic attack 62
Trauma 27–34
  blood loss 138
  cervical spine injury 133–4,
    138–9
  conscious patient 138–9
  dental floss 96
  emergency treatment in
    hospital 133–49
  facial injury see facial injury
  fixed appliances 107
  head injury 141–4
  history 27
  iatrogenic see iatrogenic
    trauma
  permanent dentition 31–4
    anterior tooth crown

fracture 33
anterior tooth root fracture
   33
completely avulsed tooth
   32–3
partially avulsed tooth 31
posterior tooth crown
   fracture 34
posterior tooth root
   fracture 34
primary dentition 29–30
removable appliances 106
soft tissues 28–9
toothbrush 96
unconscious patient 137
Traumatic ulcer 40
Traumatized denture
   granuloma 15
Tumours 22–3

facial-pain causing 13, 125
   investigations 125

Ulceration 40–3
   aphthous 41–3
   malignant 41
   recurrent 41–3
   traumatic 40
Uncemented bridge retainer 85
Uncemented crown 83
Uncemented post crown 84–5
Unconscious patient 56–62, 137

Vincent's infection (acute
   necrotising ulcerative
   gingivitis) 43, 94–6
Vitamin B_{12} deficiency 48, 155

White patches 50–2